Praise for *Love Is the Strongest Medicine*

"Laughter heals, music is medicine, and each patient is a unique, beautiful soul. These are truths we in the medical community sometimes lose track of in the routines of patient care. . . . Love Is the Strongest Medicine *will stay with you long after you close its cover."*

— **Daniel Amen, M.D.**, founder of the Amen Clinics, 10-time *New York Times* best-selling author, and "the most popular psychiatrist in America" (*The Washington Post*)

"Steven Eisenberg is a doctor who understands that health is just as much spiritual as physical. Love Is the Strongest Medicine *puts music, laughter, and heart front and center, and the results are magical."*

— **Mark Hyman, M.D.**, director of the Cleveland Clinic Center for Functional Medicine and #1 *New York Times* best-selling author of *Food: What the Heck Should I Eat?*

"Dr. Steven's strengths as an oncologist are forged in patient relationships that fill him with compassion, faith, commitment, grief, and joy. He has our stories and lessons etched on his heart."

— **Kris Carr**, *New York Times* best-selling author and Cancer Thriver

"If you are seeking a way to bring positive energy and healing into your own life or that of a parent, child, friend, or partner who is going through a dark time—read this beautiful, soul-healing book."

— **Dr. Kellyann Petrucci**, *New York Times* best-selling author of *Dr. Kellyann's Bone Broth Diet*, host of the PBS special *21 Days to a Slimmer, Younger You*

"Love Is the Strongest Medicine *is a story of learning to be present, connected, and expressive not just with the people we love, but with everyone in our orbit. I defy anyone to come away from this book without feeling motivated to change another person's life for the better. Eisenberg's enthusiasm is honest and infectious."*

— **JJ Virgin**, nutrition, fitness, and mindset expert and *New York Times* best-selling author of *The Virgin Diet, Sugar Impact Diet,* and *Miracle Mindset*

"In an industry largely focused on treating the sick and managing the gravely ill, Dr. Steven chooses to focus on what it's like to live life to the fullest. He is the doctor we all hope to have when we are ill— intelligent, optimistic, and compassionate. His book is a must read!"

— **Gautam Gulati**, **M.D.**, founder and CEO of The Unusual Cos, Adjunct Professor at Johns Hopkins Carey Business School

"Every doctor, nurse, patient, and family member can learn from Dr. Eisenberg's creative focus on the men and women in his care rather than on their disease. He partners with and empowers his patients to choose their own paths and shape their own futures, and does it all while singing his heart out."

— **Daniel Kraft**, **M.D.**, founder and chair of Exponential Medicine, faculty chair of medicine of Singularity University

"Dr. Eisenberg's unique experiences and the amazing lessons he takes from them evolve into a great resource for surviving cancer without losing your true being."

— **Partha Nandi**, **M.D.**, CEO and creator of the Emmy-winning *Ask Dr. Nandi* show and international best-selling author of *Ask Dr Nandi*

"Each of us intuitively knows that body and spirit are intimately intertwined. Love Is the Strongest Medicine *puts that intuition into practice as Dr. Steven Eisenberg helps his patients focus on what they love, not what they fear. I couldn't put it down!"*

— **Craig Shoemaker**, comedian and transformational leader

"Dr. Eisenberg looks at the cancer experience through multiple lenses: as a patient, a physician, a sherpa, and an artist. Thanks to his candid and sensitive approach, his readers will gain invaluable insights as they, or their loved ones, face major life challenges."

— **Alex Jadad**, **M.D.**, **Ph.D.**, healer, philosopher, educator, innovator, advocate, and founder and chairman of Beati Inc.

"Dr. Eisenberg is one of our greatest storytelling physicians . . . an insatiably expressive and creative soul . . . and a wise, compassionate, and optimistic healer. His debut book will enchant millions."

— **Michael Fishman**, founder, Consumer Health Summit

LOVE
IS THE
STRONGEST
MEDICINE

LOVE
IS THE
STRONGEST
MEDICINE

*Notes from a Cancer Doctor on
Connection, Creativity, and Compassion*

DR. STEVEN EISENBERG
with JANA MURPHY

HAY HOUSE, INC.
Carlsbad, California • New York City
London • Sydney • New Delhi

Published in the United States by: Hay House, Inc.: www.hayhouse
.com® • **Published in Australia by:** Hay House Australia Pty. Ltd.: www
.hayhouse.com.au • **Published in the United Kingdom by:** Hay House UK,
Ltd.: www.hayhouse.co.uk • **Published in India by:** Hay House Publishers
India: www.hayhouse.co.in

Cover design: Howie Severson • *Interior design:* Nick C. Welch

This book was written to provide helpful guidance and encouragement to anyone who is dealing with or supporting a loved one with cancer. It is not intended as, nor should it be used as, a guideline for any diagnostic or treatment purpose. Medical decisions should be made in consultation with a personal physician, and no book is a substitute for that relationship. In the event you use any of the information in this book for yourself, the author and the publisher assume no responsibility for your actions.

The events, places, and conversations in this book have been re-created from the author's memory of real-world situations, and the chronology of some events has been compressed. Names and identifying details of individual patients have been changed to protect their privacy.

Cataloging-in-Publication Data is on file at the Library of Congress

Hardcover ISBN: 978-1-4019-6089-6
E-book ISBN: 978-1-4019-6090-2
Audiobook ISBN: 978-1-4019-6091-9

10 9 8 7 6 5 4 3 2 1
1st edition, May 2021

Printed in the United States of America

To Julie
For showing me the beauty, meaning,
and steadfast nature of love

CONTENTS

FOREWORD

The first time I met Steven Eisenberg, we sat together at a medical innovation conference, talking about science, medicine, and of course music. I was working on a new keyboard solo for an album with Joe Perry, founding lead guitarist of Aerosmith, and he wanted to hear it—not someday, but then and there. We put our heads together, craning towards the same tiny bud-sized speaker. He listened and grinned and drummed his fingers and said something corny like *Rock on!* We both laughed until a fellow conference-goer glanced our way with a look that said, *What is up with those guys?*

What was up was this: One minute we were strangers—a neuroscientist and an oncologist at a meeting in suit jackets and work mode. The next we were like a couple of childhood pals, sitting by a campfire, sharing the kind of quietly important moment that makes a memory or cements a friendship.

Music is like that. It comes into our consciousness, evokes powerful shared emotions, and bonds us together. Does anyone ever listen to Otis Redding sing "Dock of the Bay" and not get a little wistful and lonely? Or fail to stand taller at Aretha Franklin's "Respect"? Responding to music's pull is wired into us in the way we process sound and the way we store memories of melody, lyric, and rhythm. The route is ancient, so old and deep in our brains that among the Alzheimer's patients I've spent much of my career studying, it's often among the last faculties to remain. A patient who can't remember her children's names or what she had for dinner may still be able to sit at a piano and play a song she's known all her life—and that little spark can be the last line of connection between her and the people who love her.

Steven himself is a bit of a bonding agent. He's disarming and charming, and he leans into whatever you have to share—whether it's music or science, joy or pain. He feels it with you and conveys with every fiber of his being that he cares. He's a person who buzzes with humanity and empathy, changing the energy of a room by being in it and seeing possibilities everywhere.

Of course, empathy alone isn't enough of a pillar to support great work, or even a great book. Our most perfect and productive efforts happen when the three elemental parts of our brains work together: energy and motivation from the prehistoric brainstem; emotion and empathy from our limbic system; and the capacity to imagine, create, and analyze from the newest and most uniquely human part of our minds, the frontal cortex. It's relatively easy to swing moment to moment at the mercy of the part that's demanding something immediate—like a hot meal, a good cry, or some form of self-expression. It's harder to get all three parts to work in concert, to coordinate the best of our capabilities and harness them into something unique and new—to be performing in mental 3-D.

Steven's book, like his personality, weaves together these three parts of who we are, giving credence to each and thereby making it immensely relatable and readable. *Love Is the Strongest Medicine* is the genuine, curious, intelligent, and lyrical story of a man who has looked at cancer from all angles—as a student, patient, family member, doctor, and thought leader in the field of oncology. Because he has dedicated the last 30 years of his life to mastering his craft and doing it with passion, empathy, and creativity, he's been learning and growing the entire time. We see it in the simple lesson of his first chapter—a highly memorable childhood admonition to never waste a second chance. We watch it evolve as Steven does, from a well-intentioned young doctor who's terrified to write his first chemotherapy orders to a physician-philosopher who lives and breathes healing and positivity. We witness the roles music plays in his life—a source of comfort, an impetus of laughter, a basis for validation, a way to communicate when nothing else is working—and see them reflected in our own lives and our own soundtracks.

By the time he hits his stride, Steven is taking us from mountaintops to treatment rooms and the quiet inner places where we keep our fears and doubts and private joys. We're considering aspects of disease and treatment that too often get pushed to the wayside. We're asking ourselves important questions about how we treat each other, what drives and replenishes us, and where we find meaning and solace and even happiness in the midst of dealing with illness and even death. We're wondering what creative endeavor might help each of us find the kind of authenticity and good will this author achieves when he decides it's okay to pull down the walls that separate his personal church and state: medicine and music.

In the field of neurology, we often think and talk about perspective. Of course there's biological perspective, in which our genes influence our actions and reactions. And recent discoveries lead us to consider the opposite angle—how our actions influence our genes. There are countless other ways we are influenced in what we see and hear and perceive. Steven's perspective is one that's enlightening and empowering, always seeking higher ground for his patients, his relationships, and himself. He demonstrates it in his commitment to living on the cutting edge of medicine, embracing (and pioneering) new diagnostic and treatment technologies, and equally in his constant mindfulness that *care* is key to health care.

This eloquent book is an invitation to shift our perspective during the frightening and intimidating cancer experience. It offers understanding, encouragement, and empowerment to anyone who's in the middle of it or supporting someone through. It's a little comfort between two covers, a love note to patients and partners, an offer of an ear bud to share Steven's soundtrack, and a seat at his campfire.

One of the concepts that's come up many times in my life is the truth that you can't author anyone else's experience. I can point my finger at the moon and say, *Look at how beautiful*, but any earthshaking realization you ever have about just how spectacular it is will have to come from inside—your eyes, your mind. What I can do, maybe, through the power of connection, is help another person be open to that experience. I believe this book will open many hearts and minds, leaving them ready to recognize that next beautiful thing.

— Rudolph Tanzi, Ph.D.

Dr. Rudolph Tanzi is the director of the Genetics and Aging Research Unit, co-director of the McCance Center for Brain Health, and vice-chair of neurology research at Massachusetts General Hospital. He is the Joseph P. and Rose F. Kennedy Professor of Neurology at Harvard Medical School and the recipient of numerous awards, including the Smithsonian American Ingenuity Award and inclusion among Time's *100 Most Influential People in the World. Dr. Tanzi is the* New York Times *best-selling author of* Super Brain, Super Genes, *and* The Healing Self *with Deepak Chopra, as well as co-author of* Decoding Darkness. *In his spare time, he composes and records his own music and plays keyboards for Joe Perry, Aerosmith, and other musicians.*

INTRODUCTION

Only when it is dark enough can you see the stars.

— Martin Luther King, Jr.

For nearly two decades, I've been telling my oncology patients, with only a little irony, *Welcome to your new normal.* There's no getting around the fact that a cancer diagnosis— for you or someone you love—is life-changing. Sometimes those changes are temporary (even though they can *feel* like they're forever). Sometimes they're indelible. Since roughly one in three of us will be diagnosed with an invasive cancer in our lifetime, and the other two will likely know someone who receives that diagnosis, it's a menace that ultimately impacts nearly everyone.

The year 2020 will go down in history as the year the pandemic monster came and rattled the cage of the world, bringing all of us challenges we weren't prepared to face. It created a new normal for everyone, redefining our peaks and valleys and relationships, what we are afraid of, and what matters most to us. It strained the medical community, and it frequently put cancer patients in the back seat, waiting for treatment, worrying about the virus, wearing masks and gloves and praying their weakened systems would be able to hold firm. Some immune systems did not, and so we had patients fighting the double whammy of COVID-19 *and* cancer. For me and my colleagues in oncology practice, and for medical personnel all over the world, it meant a new rhythm and intensity and higher stakes than ever.

The menace of a world pandemic also made telemedicine not just a theoretical possibility but the way things get done. Many patients in my oncology practice are immunocompromised, so if an individual doesn't need chemo or lab work, we keep them home if we can. There's been a surprising upside to this for me because it's a new way to connect—just when I thought I'd learned them all. There's nothing quite like getting a view inside each other's homes to make us feel closer. Through telemedicine calls I've gotten to meet my patients' pets, admire family photos, and peek at their potted plants. I've asked some to get closer so I can scan the books on the coffee table or to show me what's for dinner (*You've got LOTS of fresh veggies in that fridge, right?*). We've laughed about unmade beds, half-done DIY projects, and family members who can't seem to help getting in the frame. On my end, I've offered up introductions to my dogs and sometimes my family, tours of my "manctuary" home office with its shag carpet, carved Buddhas, lava lamp, religious and self-help books, my guitar, and the self-portrait I painted with my hands (no brushes!) for an assignment in college.

One patient asked about my most prized possession, and that gave me a chance to open the desk drawer that's brimming with treasured mementos. It's got thank-you notes and poems, postcards from remission vacations, candles and glass figurines, and memorial prayer cards from patients and families. And it has selfies—me with my tall shock of curly hair, usually making faces; my patients with even crazier faces, or sweet smiles, or shy grins. Sometimes we're leaning into each other or holding hands; sometimes we've got our tongues sticking out or our thumbs up; sometimes one of us is bald and thin after going through the gantlet of chemotherapy and coming out the other side.

I like to think of each of those photos and gifts as a little love story. Each one commemorates a relationship that is more and deeper than doctor–patient to me. In medicine, doctors care for patients, sure, but if we're doing it right, that care goes beyond diagnosis and treatment—into the territory of caring the way we do for our fathers and mothers, brothers and sisters, aunts, uncles, cousins, and friends.

Unfortunately, that's not always the case and not always possible. We live in a world where the practice of medicine is conducted at arm's length, through machines, across the Internet, and within models where an invisible moat divides us. It often feels like doctors are on one side of that moat and patients are on the other, and as complex matters of insurance, approvals, corporate policy, and even politics find their way into hospitals and exam rooms, the moat widens, sometimes until it feels like a chasm between people who should be relying on each other and working together. There may be no field where we need each other more, where that chasm does more damage, than in oncology. Cancer patients come to their doctors at their most vulnerable. They wonder how they're going to get up each day. How they're going to tell their families about their prognosis. Why they should subject themselves to brutal treatments or daunting odds. Whether they dare hope for a cure.

It all demands a relationship, not a service, between doctor and patient.

We know this is true in our hearts and minds, but we also know it to be true in documentable terms. Studies have proven that strong, empathic engagement between doctors and their patients increases patients' willingness to report symptoms and concerns. That in turn improves diagnostic accuracy. Empathy increases patient engagement and compliance. Some studies suggest it even improves survival rates. Connection is a powerful intangible—like family, or love, or hope.

So how can a doctor bring connection into the room in the small, often intense increments of time we have with our patients? Often it's through surprising secret tools— things like laughter, empathy, and music.

There's notable science to each. Laughter has been shown to reduce stress and improve immune function. Empathy strengthens patients' ability to cope with difficult treatments and eases suffering during end-of-life care. And music—wow—studies show music can lower patient anxiety levels during invasive procedures, ease the nausea caused by chemotherapy, decrease pain perception, and inspire feelings of peace and spirituality. And that's just the medical stuff. On a personal level, listening to and making music together creates a sense of shared experience and kinship. It fires up emotional receptors that otherwise remain dormant. It is an honest, authentic shortcut to connection.

This book came about after I started a blog called *Daily Dose* in 2017, swearing I would write *something* every day. I'm not sure what I thought those somethings would be, but it turns out most of them tie back to a few key themes in my work and my life—the power of music, the inner strength in each cancer warrior, the beauty of the here and now, and, at the bedrock of my beliefs, the healing power of connection. The blog's been a place to explore my feelings and frustrations and to freely indulge in my fondness for mnemonic devices. A place where *CPR* means *compassion, presence, resilience.*

I wish I could say I always had these priorities in line, but we all have to start somewhere, to learn through steps and stops and setbacks. My own journey into medicine starts with me bleeding all over the pavement on a leafy suburban street, wanders through periods of doubt and frustration, briefly veers into despair, and ultimately puts me on an ever-more-beautiful winding road. Here I have the privilege of meeting and treating people who challenge and inspire, who teach and learn, who suffer and heal, live and sometimes die. There's hope around every bend on this road, and even when there's heartbreak, there's love—the strongest medicine.

CHAPTER 1

WANNA BE STARTIN' SOMETHIN'

I had a moment.
Triple lindy,
Broken bones,
Brain edema.
Dead?
Not yet.
It was the right place,
The right time,
To get a second chance.

— *DAILY DOSE, OCTOBER 26, 2017*

I live in California now, but sometimes when I visit Pennsylvania, I go back to the corner of Dillon Road and Keisel Lane, look at the pavement and think, *This is where your life almost ended.*

It was a moment in my childhood that likely put me on the path to becoming the doctor I am today. I was 13 years old, riding my bike to meet a friend for a tennis match. I was making big, swooping arcs as I rolled down Keisel, building up speed, pumping the pedals. When I reached the intersection at Dillon, I swung out into the street.

The car—a red station wagon driven by a woman who probably still sees me in her nightmares—hit me head on. My bike folded and my body kept moving, slamming into and shattering the windshield, falling back onto the hood, then dropping to the pavement.

I was in and out of consciousness, frantic efforts to save me coming through in hazy glimpses—neighbors crowding in the street; my mother looking down at me with tears streaming down her face; a paramedic yelling *Puncture wound!* and *Cut the pants!* I remember a flash of being in the ambulance. It's a jumble I'll never get fully sorted.

My injuries were grim. My left ear dangled. My skin was lacerated from jaw to collarbone. The pinkie on my left hand was nearly severed. My right leg was broken, the tibia grotesquely piercing the skin. But the most serious injury wasn't visible. My brain had suffered a traumatic impact and was swelling more with every passing hour. This was the wound the doctors told my parents to worry about. If I could survive that, everything else would heal.

What I remember most vividly of those first traumatic days is not my pain or even my fear. It's the kind eyes of the plastic surgeon peering out at me from between the top of his surgical mask and the bottom of the bright circle of light from his headlamp, and the steady, reassuring drone of his voice as he talked me through the hours it took to stitch my ear back to my scalp and resecure the wayward pinkie to its rightful position.

"Stay calm, Stevie," he said.

"You're doing great."

"So you must be in the eighth grade . . . "

"This is going well."

"You're going to be fine, good as new."

Dr. Kodsi's even-keeled kindness was generous and calming, especially at a time when my guts were churning with panic and anxiety and I was desperately wishing to turn back time and somehow avoid the accident. Fat, hot tears rolled down my face while he made one tiny, meticulous stitch after another. I focused on his eyes and his soft, steady voice. Like everything from those first days after the accident, I remember the hours we spent together in a reel of cobbled-together snippets—willing myself to be perfectly still, wincing at the throbbing pain in my leg, gazing up at the light of that headlamp.

I spent a month in the hospital, first flat in bed in a full-leg cast, then in a wheelchair, and eventually progressing to hobbling up and down the halls on crutches. Through much of that time, I suffered from a condition called *expressive aphasia*, caused by the swelling in my brain interfering with my ability to speak. I could think of what I wanted to say, but I couldn't get the words out. So I found a different way. I know now that speech and song come from different centers in the brain, but at the time all I knew was that even though I couldn't string together simple lines like *My leg hurts*, or *I'm thirsty*, or *How bad are the scars?* I had no trouble singing the lyrics of my favorite songs. My parents brought my cassette tapes and player and I quickly adapted to singing to express and entertain myself. I sang Michael Jackson's "Wanna Be Startin' Somethin'" during physical therapy, Prince's "Little Red Corvette" to make the nurses laugh, and a woeful version of Bob Marley's "Redemption Song" the first time I saw my wrecked face.

I think my mom deliberately kept my reflection out of my sight for as long as she could manage, probably hoping I would hurry up and heal before I saw the worst of it. But somebody sent me a get-well card with mirrored paper inside, and that's where I caught my first glimpse of the damage. My face was a patchwork of black stitches, jaggedly marring my cheek and my jaw and marching down my

3

neck. I thought I looked like Frankenstein. I looked away, and kept singing. I was developing a different, deeper kind of connection with music while it was my only means of verbal communication—a relationship that's stayed with me ever since.

That first moment of clarity that my body was not the same and would likely never be is one I often go back to, a touchstone in my connection with my oncology patients today. So often, having to accept the outward signs of illness—scars, hair loss, and other changes that physically mark the fight against cancer—is one of the struggles of being in treatment. When your private pain is out there for the world to see, that's a different kind of unfairness from living with disease in the first place. It demands we face the identity issues that go hand-in-hand with a serious illness: *How am I different? How much will this change me and my relationships?*

It's hard for a 13-year-old to put anything in perspective, let alone something as monumental as wrecking your own body from head to toe. As the worst of my injuries began to heal, I became obsessed with my messed-up face—the clear-as-day proof that I was irrevocably altered by the accident. That's when my father decided it was time to tell me the rest of the story. He sat beside me in our backyard one afternoon, both of us looking out at his blooming garden rather than at one another. We'd always done our bonding outside—playing baseball, football, and Frisbee; pulling weeds from the flower and vegetable beds where he'd earned his neighborhood nickname of Barry Greenthumb. I hadn't thrown a ball or pulled a weed in weeks by then. I'd come home from the hospital in a deep funk, taken up sleeping late and eating on the couch, and avoided mirrors as much as possible. I guess he thought I'd wallowed long enough. He let out a big sigh and then told me how he remembered the accident.

With quiet detachment he recounted the day, my mother's sobbing phone call, the frantic rush to the hospital, the way the medical team had triaged my wounds, dealing with each in order of urgency. He told me how he'd tried to process each update rationally, letting the physician side of him take control, and how my mom had been shocked and terrified. He explained that when it seemed the worst was over, when each wound had been inspected and assessed and given due attention, they'd gone home, physically and mentally exhausted.

When the phone rang in the middle of the night, he said he'd pounced on it, knowing no good news comes from the hospital in the wee hours. It was a nurse from the ICU. "Steven has stopped breathing," she said. "We're intubating him. You should come now."

With his composure starting to waver, Dad recounted hearing a voice in the background, saying "We're losing him," and leaping to his feet, already moving toward the door. He could picture the medical team working frantically over my battered body.

Before my parents could make their way back to the hospital, the doctors and nurses brought me back and stabilized me. Mom and Dad considered it a miracle.

"We thought we were going to lose you forever," my father said in the garden.

We sat with that for a minute, but he wasn't finished. "Your face is going to heal, Steven," he said. "One day soon you'll hardly be able to tell you had those stitches. I want you to try to stop worrying about that. The important thing is that you're still here."

I was mulling this over, still not feeling very lucky, when he added, "Getting a second chance is a gift, son. Don't ever take your life for granted."

It's been decades since the accident and since that moment when my usually reserved father let his guard down and gave me a piece of advice that stuck. From that day until this one, my existence has in many ways become an exercise in embracing the gift of life. I was never the same kid after the accident as I was before. I was moodier and more rebellious at school. I was quicker to say what I really thought instead of what I thought I ought to say. I was more devoted than ever to music and the always-changing roster of bands I was forming and joining and quitting.

When I had trouble sleeping because I couldn't shake the trauma of the accident and its aftermath, sometimes I'd calm myself by imagining the kind eyes and reassuring voice of the surgeon who'd sewn me back together. I could picture the halo from the light he was using while he stitched, remember sensing the movement of his hands but not feeling them against my skin. In those moments I started to think maybe a doctor was who I wanted to be—a doctor who could bring calm reassurance and even hope into the room, who could gently steer patients back toward life.

In the years that followed, I frequently found myself on the fringes of the medical profession—volunteering at a nursing home and in an ER waiting room, hanging out in my dad's medical office, exploring the possibilities of the mind–body connection through yoga and meditation, and pulling each self-help book from my parents' bookshelf in turn, flipping through the pages and trying to figure out how it all related to my own teenaged life.

My 13-year-old self healed and grew, and when the time came, I chose medical school and then, eventually, oncology—a field devoted to the art and science of creating second chances.

Bearing witness to patients' struggles, victories, relationships, and discoveries as they embrace their second chances and, sometimes, as they confront mortality, is both a burden and a privilege. It is an opportunity to learn and grow and marvel at the power of human connection. And it is, like the accident and my recovery before it, a powerful gift that reminds me every day of my father's admonition: "Don't ever take your life for granted."

CHAPTER 2

MY WAY

You may lose.
But don't lose yourself.
You may feel abandoned.
But don't abandon yourself.
You may not know the answer.
But know who you are.

— *DAILY DOSE*, MAY 14, 2020

The question every oncologist gets asked again and again is, *Isn't it depressing?*

The answer is that it can be, that once in a while it stomps on your heart. But focusing on the hardest days misses the point. Oncology allows me the privilege of being useful to patients and their families, of getting to know them, of being with them during some of the lowest lows and highest highs of their lives. It is personal, emotional, and full of moments when hope, faith, love, forgiveness, and family win the day. Facing down even the distant specter of death in the form of cancer—no matter how treatable—can be transformative. It makes us think about who and what matters most to us, what we want from our lives, and how we want to spend our days. Witnessing that process and the surprising, inspiring ways it plays out brings joy and purpose to my days.

It took a long time to get to this place. After my accident, I had a vague sense that I wanted to be a doctor, that maybe I could do for other people what Dr. Kodsi had done for me—offering comfort and healing and hope when I felt irrevocably broken.

Of course, I also wanted to be a rock star. I founded and played in so many bands I lost count. Among them was a synth-pop duo called The Slew, a British punk trio we named The Killas (no matter that none of us was British), an alternative group called The Toothpicks, and a mixed-genre quartet dubbed Crab Meat Copenhagen. Rarely was I ever *not* in a band. Writing songs and collaborating with bandmates and playing for anybody who would listen was an integral part of my identity.

I also dreamed I'd one day get "the call" from Lorne Michaels, asking me to audition for *Saturday Night Live*. He'd have heard one of the cassette tapes of jokes I used to record (far too many of them at the expense of my little sister) or, later, seen me doing stand-up in some dive bar. He'd say, "Stevie, you're just what *SNL* needs right now."

I didn't know it then, but the one thing all my passions shared was that at their core they were ways of making connections—of building bonds in a hurry. I was still learning how central this process would be in my life. It wasn't until I was in medical school that I started to see just how crucial connection might be in a physician's career—especially that of an oncologist.

♡

When you set out to go to medical school, there are two parallel paths from which to choose. The more traditional route is becoming an M.D.—doctor of medicine. The road somewhat less traveled is pursuing a D.O.—doctor of osteopathic medicine. Both are equally rigorous—four years of medical school and a residency—but the M.D. focuses first on the diagnosis and treatment of ailments. The D.O. is a little more holistic, presuming that the body naturally trends toward being healthy and pushing the physician to focus on the whole patient rather than any specific condition. As a yoga-doing, arts-loving, self-help junkie in my early 20s, I chose the D.O. route and enrolled at the Philadelphia College of Osteopathic Medicine.

It was at PCOM that I met one of the great mentors of my life. Emanuel Fliegelman, who insisted students call him Uncle Manny, taught obstetrics, gynecology, and various courses about human sexuality. His classes were always packed.

On my first day of medical school, Dr. Fliegelman gestured toward the entrance of the lecture hall and warned, with no small amount of drama, "Do not pass through these doors without the Ten Cs." And then he laid out his plan for our betterment, one C at a time. He told us to be compassionate and caring, approaching each patient's world from a place of respect. He told us to make contact, with something as simple as a touch on the hand or a pat on the back. He emphasized both a focus on competence based on learning over a lifetime and the creativity of thinking outside the exam room box. He encouraged us to communicate, starting with listening with our full attention.

Sitting in my uncomfortable chair, I stopped squirming after his second point. This was not what I'd expected in my first lecture. This wasn't data or disease or anatomy or diagnosis. These were words to live by. By the tenth point, I was ready to follow this man anywhere and take his advice on anything. He was the living embodiment of compassion in connecting with patients that I'd hoped to find.

This is what I want to be, I thought, looking up at the balding man with the iron-grey beard and bright eyes—his face seemingly always on the verge of a smile and a wink.

Starting with that first encounter, Uncle Manny gradually and profoundly changed my life. He was an accomplished physician, a generous teacher, and a kind man. He was also a bit of a ham (we were kindred spirits in that). He said he loved to lecture, that he should have to pay to do it for all the joy and euphoria it gave him. He was dramatic, open, loving, and oh-so-funny—that last quality decidedly not a common one among the med school faculty.

Dr. Fliegelman set the course of my intentions and attitudes as a young doctor, and he became a dear friend. For years after med school, whenever I faced a professional crisis or question, I'd call and he'd answer and help me work it out.

One of his signature encouragements for his students was *Be a beacon for compassion.*

Sometimes it seemed like Dr. Fliegelman's good nature was contagious. I remember him joking with the expectant mothers during my obstetrics rotation, naturally, gently putting them at ease. One of these patients, who was having the first twins I'd assist with, seemed to be playing along with him in trying to put *me* at ease. As I nervously monitored her contractions, I asked the expectant mom what she envisioned for her family's future and then if she'd thought of any names for her soon-to-be-born boys.

"I was thinking of naming them Orangello and Lemongello," she said brightly. I looked up from my chart, searching her face for some sign she was joking, and she let me hang for several seconds before reaching across the bedrail to the dinner tray that had inadvertently been brought to her room. She jiggled the edge, and the bowl of Jell-O on the corner jiggled as well. Then she winked and burst out laughing.

"Don't worry, honey," she said. "We're both going to be fine."

I'm not sure who was really taking care of who that day.

It wasn't until much later that I'd learn laughing actually increases a person's pain threshold, but I did catch on quickly to the fact that a well-placed joke could ratchet down the anxiety during even a potentially intense medical interaction.

"Childbirth should be a joyful event," Dr. Fliegelman had told us. That night, it was.

♡

Of course, not all professors can be warm and cuddly. Some are imposing, even borderline scary. John Simelaro, for example, with his thick black hair, square jaw, and strong build, looked, walked, and talked like a middle-aged Rocky Balboa. He was a brilliant, passionate doctor and teacher who carried his South Philly heritage loud and proud. When Dr. S. spoke, his thick accent gave everything a tinge of "Yo, Adrian," even when his words were straight-up medical jargon. He was a presence, and his students were so intimidated by him that we secretly called him the Godfather. We were also eager to impress him. Here was a doctor who advocated for his patients like nobody's business. He treated them like his big South Philly *famiglia,* and if you were one of his residents, it was assumed that you too would respect and watch over his beloved family.

During my first year of residency, I was working in Dr. S.'s clinic when I met Barb, an elderly patient with advanced lung cancer in addition to COPD (chronic obstructive pulmonary disease). I was shadowing Dr. S., and after he greeted Barb and introduced me, he held her hand, asked about her family, then her symptoms, and then began his exam.

"Stevie," he said, "you should listen to these lungs, if Barb doesn't mind."

"Of course he can," she said. "Somebody ought to get some use out of them."

Barb's breathing was a jumble of wheezes and crackles, and it was an effort for her to take just a few deep breaths for me. I knew from her chart that she'd nearly exhausted the treatments available to her. She was at the end of six rounds of palliative chemo aimed at keeping her comfortable and giving her more time with her family. Even with the treatment, her condition was deteriorating.

You'd never have known it from her attitude. Barb was boisterous and flirty, wearing a bright red knit hat and winking at Dr. S. while I examined her. Despite her diagnosis and her treatment, she'd refused to give up cigarettes—coming in from the cold with the scent of tobacco still clinging to her clothes.

Dr. S. inquired about her diet, her meds, and her sleep. He nudged her, probably for the umpteenth time, to quit smoking. He asked if she had anyone to check in on her at home. Then he leaned close and asked if there was anything else he could do for her.

I was learning every minute about how to really care for the person on my exam table.

During morning report we talked about Barb's case, and the next time she came to clinic, I saw her on my own. Some students shrank away from her, not sure how to handle this brash, noncompliant, dying woman, but I was thrilled to see her. She may have posed a medical challenge, but she was a pistol—quick and funny, with a big laugh and an easy confidence implying that after nearly seven decades of life lived fully, she had no regrets.

I listened to her weakening heart and lungs, then tweaked her anti-nausea meds in hopes of making her more comfortable. I asked about her family. Barb had five grown children and a dozen grandchildren. She listed all their names. She told me how her neighborhood had become so crime-ridden that her little house was flanked on either side by abandoned properties, but that she wasn't scared to stay. She said her favorite meal was chicken parmesan and her favorite song had been the same since it was released in 1969: Frank Sinatra's "My Way." She even sang me a verse, stopping to catch her breath before the chorus.

That night as I walked home to my little studio apartment, punch drunk with exhaustion, I sang "My Way" in the street. I fell asleep hoping my patient was also snug in her bed, slumbering comfortably.

♡

My whole life music had been helping me cope with the things I was dealing with. I'd been writing lyrics for as long as I could remember, scribbling them on napkins, on loose-leaf paper, in piano practice books. Making sense of words and putting them to music helped me make sense of everything else. In medical school, the margins of my notes were littered with half-baked lyrics. One day we learned about a procedure called a sympathectomy, which involves cutting or blocking a nerve. The minute I heard the term, lyrics started swimming in my head. *I don't need your sympathy—I'm getting a sympathectomy,* and *You don't have to feel for me. I've had my sympathectomy.* Who would have thought even medical terminology would offer infinite phrasing opportunities?

For some students sleep was the antidote to the stress of the program. It was such a scarcity, they took nearly every non-studying, non-hospital minute to close their eyes and just rest. Others partied in their off-hours or tried to maintain fraying relationships with partners who often had a hard time accepting that residency is a 100-hour-a-week commitment—sometimes more.

Music was what got me through. I was in downtown Philadelphia, surviving on cheesesteaks and bottles of Ensure nipped from hospital fridges, but on the nights I was off, I'd practice my guitar (an instrument I'd picked up after college because it was infinitely more portable than my parents' piano), work out my lyrics, and play a few songs at any club or café that would have me. When the going got toughest near the end of school and I started to feel crushed by the pressure, I packed up my battered guitar and drove into New York for an open casting call for *Rent*. I waited in line for hours before my turn to perform—as if there was a chance in hell I had the professional skills and experience to land a Broadway role (or the time to commit to one if I got it!). As soon as I was done, I drove back to Philly and hit the books again. Somehow the experience made me feel better about everything. Just as I'd done in the weeks following my bicycle accident, I'd been able to use music to push through.

I was beginning to get the hang of feeling responsible for my own patients, gaining a little confidence, when I got a 1 A.M. call from the emergency room. This didn't necessarily constitute an emergency, because everyone at the hospital knows you can call a resident at any hour with any question, no matter how small. I answered groggily, wondering what minutiae was cutting into my precious five hours of downtime. I snapped awake though, when the ER resident said, "We've got one of your patients here, and she's circling the drain."

It was Barb. I was so disgusted with the resident's flippant comment that I stomped across the on-call room where I'd been trying to grab a couple hours' sleep and slammed the door on the way out to the ER. I found her alone in her room, gasping for air. She reached for my hand and pled for relief, her thick Philly accent wavering as she said, "I don't want to do this anymore."

I knew she wouldn't have to—her hands were cool, her breathing irregular and punctuated by too-long pauses. She was approaching death. I could sign her over to hospice, but I worried she might continue to suffer for hours before someone could take charge of her case. So I admitted her, ordered a morphine drip, and worked to make her comfortable. Morphine is a small miracle for patients who reach this end stage of life. It not only masks physical pain but takes away the feeling of air hunger that causes so much suffering. As Barb's strained breathing started to ease, I called her family.

From her bed, Barb whispered, "Thanks, hon," and patted my hand.

I was still learning, am always learning, how to find my place in scenes like the sad one that followed. Barb's children arrived, sorrowful but not surprised. They gathered around her bed, held her hands, spoke softly. She consoled them as best she could. I came and went from the room, trying to keep to the corners and only approach Barb when she was in distress. At some point, her son cued up "My Way" on a portable CD player, and we all listened.

Barb smiled and said, "They're playing my song."

When Barb died that morning, she drifted off between breaths, a quiet passing for a woman who had lived loud.

I left the family to spend a few last quiet moments with their mother, realizing as I checked the time that I was late for morning rounds—a cardinal sin for a resident. Nearly doubled over with anxiety and terrified of how I'd be received, I raced through the halls. When I came crashing in on my group, 15 minutes late, Dr. S. glared at me and demanded to know what possible excuse I could have.

Stammering, I told him about Barb's case, her family, and her passing. When I stopped talking, all the interns (including me) stared at the floor, waiting for the inevitable, blistering rebuke.

Instead I got a benediction.

"Stevie, you've got a good heart," Dr. S. said kindly. Then he turned his attention to the group, raising his voice and resuming his tough-guy inflection. "Don't you *ever* leave a dying patient," he said. "It's your job to be there, to take care of the family. That's what compassion is, and you cannot and should not be a doctor without compassion."

I was stunned, and sad, and proud. For the first time I felt like maybe I was worthy of being part of Dr. S.'s *famiglia*— that when my patient was in need, there might be a little sliver of Rocky in me too.

After that, I began noticing how strongly I felt drawn to my oncology patients, and, ironically after Barb's passing, how hopeful I felt that I might be able to contribute to their treatments, speed their recoveries, or ease their suffering. I'd never wanted to be a surgeon, but I'd considered a number of other medical specialties. It was in oncology, though, that I found myself building relationships, meeting families, hearing patient stories, and somehow feeling like what I had to offer was most worthwhile.

I couldn't have known then that I was choosing a field where hopeful advances were coming, where the rate of survivorship of all cancers was on the rise, where the percentage of patients who *live* would steadily rise from around 50 percent to nearly 70 percent. Or that the kinds of relationships I wanted to build with my patients might one day be instrumental not only in getting many of them diagnosed and through treatment, but also in them getting on with their lives as survivors.

Barb's case had shown me a devastatingly callous side of medicine—the tired ER intern coldly dismissing the suffering of a dying patient. I'm sure it was a survival mechanism for that guy, but it was a side of the work I was determined to avoid. Uncle Manny had taught me that compassion was the key to consistently doing the right thing by my patients. Choosing oncology would mean choosing relationships, getting close, learning each patient's story. It would be personal and meaningful. It was exactly the right path.

♡

Around the same time I decided to pursue oncology, I also started thinking about making a different kind of commitment. I was tired of playing the old restrung right-hand guitar I'd salvaged from my parents' attic. Paul McCartney played a true lefty. So did Kurt Cobain. I was a left-handed, guitar-playing songwriter too. I got a little bit obsessed about it, calling and checking music stores every few days until the clerk at a place on Lancaster Avenue answered and said, "We just have one, but it's a beauty." I went down and played it—and fell in love. It was an Ovation Legend acoustic-electric, made of spruce with an ebony fretboard in a color called Cherry Burst. I had about $1,000 to my name, and I spent more than half that day on the guitar. I felt elevated from poser to rock star just by carrying the thing around. I went home wondering, as I often did, if there was some way I could find a confluence of these two things—music and medicine—that made me feel like I had a mission in the world.

Of course it was already there, in bonding with Barb over a favorite song and letting out the frustrations of the day by singing my heart out along the streets of Philadelphia. It was there in the way I hunched over that new guitar and tried to work out just the right melody and chords for the sympathectomy song. Music was making me a more caring doctor, and being a doctor was making me a more passionate songwriter.

Learning to pour my emotions between those two vessels kept either from overflowing.

In the world of cancer care, no matter from what angle you're experiencing it, the things you're passionate about can serve the same function the music vessel does for me. They can help you tune in or tune out, balance your fears and hopes, and remember who you are and what you're all about. I've had patients who find this other vessel in poetry, carpentry, knitting, sketching, yoga, meditation, volunteering, baking, stargazing, walking, and just sitting by the ocean. It doesn't matter what it is; it matters how it makes you feel. Focus on your breathing, on if your fists or jaw are clenched, on whether you can get swept away by your activity. We all need to be able to get away from the pressures of our lives, especially in times of stress and illness. If you're coping with cancer, now is not the time to give up the things that make you feel normal and creative and immersed. Keep them close and use them often.

CHAPTER 3

LET LOVE RULE

HOPE:
Hold On, Pain Ends

— *Daily Dose*, May 15, 2017

Even though there are doctors, scientists, and statisticians devoted to understanding and predicting disease trends, diagnoses, and prognoses, dealing with cancer is always an individual journey. There are no hard-and-fast rules. The ways patients present, the ways they cope, the ways they choose to pursue treatment, and the ways they respond to it are all deeply personal. I was lucky to learn very early in my career that I should never make assumptions.

On day one of my fellowship at Georgetown University's Lombardi Comprehensive Cancer Center, the program director leveled his gaze at the seven new fellows, cocked his finger at us, and flatly stated, "Chemotherapy is a loaded gun." He paused and scanned our faces. "It is far too easy to kill the patient along with the cancer."

Each of the fellows at the table was eager to be a warrior in the fight against cancer, but we were also scared to death. We glanced around at one another, shuffled our feet, drummed our fingers, and tried not to look like deer in the headlights. Nobody ever wants to hear the words *easy to kill the patient*—least of all a group of newly minted fellows taking their first baby steps in the oncology department. We were hoping to *save* lives.

In our first weeks at the hospital, we saw the truth behind the director's warning. Sometimes it felt like disease was only half of what was harming our patients—and the other half was treatment. At first glance choosing oncology seems to be about giving comfort—and a lot of the time it is—but I was quickly learning that sometimes I had to hand out pain instead. I had to ask patients to buy in to going to war against the cancer in their bodies. *I've got this pill/infusion and it's going to make you feel like hell . . . but it's going to root out the cancer and give you back your life.* Inevitably, the metaphor of the loaded gun stuck with me, with chemo as its ammunition.

Every day we were learning about different types of chemotherapy, and every day we saw treatment's walking wounded. Patients with painful neuropathy in their feet. Patients whose heart muscles were weakened. Patients whose white blood cells had been blasted so effectively that they could no longer fight off even the mildest infection. We learned to despise certain drugs—some of which have since been improved or replaced and some of which have not—but we still had to rely on them.

We were constantly asking, *Can I give this person one more bullet? Should I?* There were so many bullets, so many things to learn, and so much to absorb about the compromises that must be made every day in oncology. The first year I was laser-focused on just not messing up. Like the other fellows, I didn't want to be the one to fire the wrong bullet, to cause any unnecessary harm. On paper we were a team of shining students from our respective medical schools; but in practice we were intimidated by the high stakes. I had taken an oath to heal and do no harm with a pure heart, but I'd had no idea it would be so complicated to adhere to it.

When I met William, one of my first patients as a resident, he was suffering from head and neck cancer, with a grapefruit-sized tumor that started in his tongue and extended through his throat. He was unable to eat or drink normally or swallow without pain, and as a likely consequence, he was rail thin. He had a deep tan and heavily etched wrinkles in his face that made him look older than his 58 years. He held his body rigid, and his pale blue eyes stayed closed an extra beat when he blinked—clear signs he was in pain. He had a brutal tumor that had spread to the lymph nodes in his neck. I couldn't help but wonder how big a bullet to the throat a man could really take.

Getting my patients engaged in dialogue was one of the few tools I knew how to use to put them at ease back then, and this was particularly challenging with William because it hurt him to speak. He stared back at me and said nothing as I reviewed his case, only nodding or shaking his head at my questions. He had come alone, and I remember wishing he had someone there to hold his hand. Since it was just the two of us, I tentatively reached out, covering his hand with mine for just a few seconds. I didn't want to intrude on his personal space, but I wanted to offer more reassurance than my words were going to be able to give.

I started with the upside—that we could help him better manage his discomfort. Then I explained the extent of the cancer we could see in his imaging studies and the options that were likely available for his treatment. I looked even younger than my 29 years, and so in addition to grappling with his diagnosis and treatment recommendations, I imagine William was wondering how old this wild-haired, gangly-legged kid in the white coat was and whether I was qualified to help him.

He didn't need to worry on that score, because every step I took as a fellow was analyzed by an A team of seasoned, expert oncologists. Before I could implement any treatment plan, I'd report William's case and my recommendations in minute detail, and my assumptions would be considered and challenged. When I presented this case to my professors and the other fellows, explaining William's condition, the relevant literature, and the treatment I'd recommend, I did it feeling the full weight of the life-and-death stakes. I also did it under the hostile scrutiny of the professor I'd come to think of as Dr. Jekyll. Each day during morning report, he was there in the front row and off to my left, seemingly lying in wait to wreck me. Many mornings just the fact of his presence made me so nervous I'd vomit in the restroom before making my presentation. He was the anti–Uncle Manny. On the day of my first report about William, I mentioned a possible medication and Jekyll bluntly interrupted, demanding, "Name all the side effects of that drug, Eisenberg. GO!" Later he heckled my pronunciation of one of the hundreds of medical terms I knew how to define but not yet how to say aloud. Even as I wrote them, I knew he'd also decimate my notes, scrawling comments like *NO!!!* and *AMATEUR* in the margins of my work. He questioned my every assessment and recommendation, and my competence along with them.

In the long run, I'd be grateful for some of this abuse, but at the time I was just trying to keep my breakfast down and stand my ground. I was trying to learn how to be a competent, compassionate oncologist, to do right by my patient. And this guy kept kicking me in the teeth.

I know now that more than anything, the fellowship professors wanted us to be better than good, better than competent. We were about to be entrusted with the care of patients battling what author and oncologist Siddhartha Mukherjee dubbed the emperor of all maladies—the many diseases we call cancer. They are varied and ancient, but they all share the single characteristic of abnormal cell growth. Sometimes that growth is plodding and silent, sometimes chaotic and obvious, but it is always unwelcome. More than any other diagnosis, it is tangled up with our personal and cultural fears and deepest vulnerabilities.

So yes, our little band of oncologists needed to be better. If we were going to make it in the field and be worthy of the work we'd signed up to do, the team at Georgetown knew they had to toughen us up.

Jekyll just had a less humane way of doing it than some of the others.

After reviewing my notes, the meticulous, thoughtful chief of head and neck cancers believed William's case was treatable. Deferring to his expertise, I wrote an order for cisplatin and fluorouracil, a potent drug combination that had demonstrated effectiveness but sometimes carried heavy side effects. I felt the weight of writing those first chemotherapy orders as if I was writing them for myself, for my mother, for my kid sister. I read and reread the paperwork a dozen times to be sure it was accurate.

♡

In an internal medicine residency, you see a lot of difficult things that people are living with—hypertension, diabetes, all kinds of diseases and disorders. But when you study oncology, you are immersed in the extremes of life and death. This was certainly the case with William, who was suffering with nearly every breath. After seeing him in clinic and examining his case, I privately thought his chemotherapy orders were probably an exercise in futility, and I readied myself to do everything possible to combat the side effects he would have to endure. Making him comfortable was the least I could do.

He was willing to try the treatment, and on the day of his first infusion, his daughter came and sat beside him. I hovered near them in my spare moments (which are few and far between for oncology fellows), trying to think of something I could do for him, coming up with nothing more than a few empty-sounding words of encouragement.

Music was still my refuge, and on days like that first day of William's treatment, when it felt like the best I had to offer was just a hard road ahead, I'd go back to my apartment, lie on the floor, and listen to Andrea Bocelli's *Sogno*, the entire album. I'd stay still, breathing deep, meditative breaths, staring at the ceiling, letting the music wash over me until I started to feel alive again. The music could reach me in a way no words ever have. It made me want to do something powerful and positive. It made me want to sing, to learn to speak Italian, to be a better doctor.

I'd often think about an admonishment from one of my PCOM professors. He told us that in medicine we'd have to either "grow or die." Listening to Bocelli made me choose to grow. When I finally felt ready to get off the floor, I'd call my fiancée, Julie, and we'd go out to eat, or I'd pack up my guitar and head to a coffee shop near my place that sometimes let me play a set.

For a while my specialty was Nirvana's "About a Girl," but I always closed with Lenny Kravitz's "Let Love Rule," and it always brought me back to my patients—not to the zombie-like devastation I'd carried home as a doctor, but to hope as someone who cared about them.

In the weeks and months that followed the initiation of William's treatment, I began to realize my hope wasn't nearly as futile as it sometimes felt. After a wretched phase when he could only get water and fluids through a gastric tube and his skin was as inflamed and raw as that of a burn victim, his grapefruit-sized tumor shrank to the size of a tennis ball. Then to a golf ball. And then to a kidney bean. Finally, to the best of our ability to detect, the cancer that had taken such an aggressive and obvious form was gone. Over a period of months, William recovered his strength. He could eat again. He could speak and sing and resume his life. His voice was gravelly and low after treatment, permanently altered. I told him I admired his new Johnny Cash–style bass, and even though he was the strong-and-silent type, William chuckled, and for just a second, he rested his hand on my back as he left the office that day.

I was awed and inspired to see the patient who'd seemed too sick for treatment amble into the clinic for his six-month follow-up. It seemed that the bullet—well-chosen, well-placed, and maybe blessed with a little luck—had blasted the cancer and spared the man.

I was also humbled. I'd made too many assumptions about William's case. My initial assessment had underestimated the possibilities. If I was going to succeed in oncology, I was beginning to realize, I'd have to learn to choose my ammunition wisely, take painstaking aim at the cancer, and willingly pull the trigger. The Lombardi director's loaded-gun warning had served its purpose, giving us a deep and abiding respect for the power of chemotherapy meds, but now it was time to embrace them as an effective weapon against disease.

William's case taught me one of the most important and impactful lessons I would ever learn as a doctor—one as blunt as the kind a kid learns by touching a hot stove: *Never* assume you *know*. Never write off anybody based on first impressions, or first scans, or past histories.

In medicine we have everything that history and diagnostic tools can offer, and we have increasingly remarkable technology and treatment regimens at our disposal. We can make solid assessments and wise recommendations. But there's a limit to how much our training, experience, and instincts can tell us. Every person is unique. For that matter, every cancer is unique too. We can categorize it by where it occurs, how it grows, and what kinds of cells it is made up of, but there are infinite variations in both the disease and the ways each person responds to it. This has become expressly clear in recent years as personalized therapies and immunologic treatments are being developed—some of them as individual as the person who receives them.

The fact is, every case has facets that can't be measured. Every time I meet a new patient or see a first scan, every time I sit down to talk with a family about options, the truth about what I *don't* know is with me. I do my best to impart that same respect for individuality to my patients. So often when families arrive, they've already taken deep dives into the Internet morass of valid and not-so-valid medical information. They've read statistics and horror stories and truths and falsehoods. Sometimes they've only heard a diagnosis from a hurried intern in an emergency room who had an incomplete snapshot of the case, who probably should have said less.

Every cancer patient has the right—maybe even the responsibility—to become informed about what they're dealing with. But the way to do that without driving yourself into web-surfing darkness is to talk with your doctor about where to find trusted sources and how to keep your case in perspective.

It's not an overstatement to say that *every* case is exceptional. William was the first of countless patients to teach me that. With that in mind, we should all agree to accept the limits of our knowledge—and then we can march into treatment together.

CHAPTER 4

WHAT A WONDERFUL WORLD

All there is to do is love one another,
Lift each other up.
Find a way to dance with even this.

— *DAILY DOSE*, APRIL 30, 2020

One of the biggest challenges of my fellowship was learning to harvest bone marrow. I'd never wanted to be a surgeon, but every hematology or oncology specialist has to master this primitive process—forcing needle into bone, twisting and guiding until you feel the telltale give of marrow, then drawing it out. As a fellow I did it day after day, week after week, honing my ability to complete the steps efficiently and effectively. I became capable, but I lacked the nuance that comes with experience. Worse, I sometimes worried my anxiety might add to the pain and stress of the process for my patients.

One morning I went into a procedure with a leukemia patient named Ken. He was in his mid-50s, a teacher with a gentle, cheerful disposition and a young family. We were both nervous (though I was trying not to show it). Ken was stretched out on his side on his hospital bed, scrubbed and prepped, his hip exposed and swabbed with iodine. After reviewing the process with him, I administered a local anesthetic. While we waited for it to take effect, I asked the question I ask most people to start getting to know them: *Do you have a favorite song?*

"'What a Wonderful World,'" he answered wryly, "even though it's not too wonderful yet today."

"Man, I love that one," I said. "What a classic." I pressed the injection area with my finger. "Do you feel that?"

"Just pressure," he said, a green light. I talked him through the hard part—making a small incision in his skin and pressing the needle deep into the pelvic bone. As I twisted the needle slowly back and forth in the area, testing resistance, feeling for the soft give of the marrow, Ken held his breath.

"Hang on, Ken. Just breathe. We're almost there. Are you okay? Am I hurting you?"

"No," he said, his muscles easing a little. "I'm okay."

"What's the first line Louis sings?" I asked.

Ken, enduring this first step in what would be a months-long fight for his health, started to quietly sing, *"I see trees of green, red roses too . . ."*

I found the spot I was looking for and asked him to take a deep breath, hold it, and then slowly exhale as I began the aspiration. I picked up the song where he'd left off, doing my best Armstrong-esque rasp, *"I see them bloom, for me and you."*

For the first time since we'd met, I heard Ken laugh, my impression apparently more froggy than jazzy. Then he raised his own voice as he joined in, *"And I think to myself, what a wonderful world."*

It was such a small thing, singing together, but I could feel this patient relax under my hands, and I could feel my own nerves ease, giving me confidence as I drew out the marrow and finished the procedure. We sang our way through it.

It would be another decade before the first studies came out confirming music can help ease patient anxiety and perception of pain during bone marrow aspiration, but I already knew it to be true.

Of course, I wasn't the first or only person seeing the power of music and art, laughter and self-expression in medicine. The idea that the arts and health are intricately entwined goes back about as far as time. In ancient Greek mythology, Apollo was the god of the arts and medicine. In the Bible, each time King Saul is plagued by the evil spirit, David plays the harp to make him feel better.

I was lucky enough to have landed in a hospital where a creative, inclusive program that formalized arts in medicine was just starting to take shape.

It was a writing expert who took the helm. Nancy Morgan was a therapeutic writing clinician, offering a unique form of therapy in which she guided patients as they wrote their stories, feelings, and experiences. Some of them wrote directly about illness, but others came at the process in their own ways, writing about family, friends, memories, gardens, or pets. Sometimes Nancy opened the door with a prompt, asking as simple a question as *What do you need?* to get the ball rolling. Any topic that put pen to paper and started getting emotions on the page was the right one, and her process was remarkably effective at helping people get at the core of what they were feeling. Fears, joys, and frustrations that were out in the open were able to be faced and dealt with. This seemingly small act—giving voice to feelings that might be buried and tangled up with illness and treatment and family dynamics—often tipped an invisible balance of power back to the writer. Defining what was going on gave them a measure of control over it.

There was no one outcome for the writing collaborators, but in my own experience, I met patients who became more able to describe their symptoms and side effects, patients who found more effective and constructive ways to relate to their families during treatment, and patients who became more assertive in the best possible way with their doctors and nurses—speaking out when they were uncomfortable or confused instead of suffering in silence. At first Nancy offered her expressive writing workshops just for patients, then also for caregivers and hospital staff. Each group, in turn, gained insight and valuable communication tools.

For me, expressive writing came naturally. I'd been doing some loose, independent form of it most of my life, writing lyrics to express my feelings and frustrations. This was the first time, though, that I understood just how much weight seemed to lift from me when I found the right words. It felt like some of my emotions spilled out onto the paper with the ink. There were plenty of emotions to manage, because an oncology fellowship is a trial by fire. There is a long learning curve to finding ways to focus on what you can do to help rather than on how much suffering you are witnessing.

While Nancy handled the writing program herself, she was soon also shepherding a comprehensive arts and humanities program, bringing musicians, painters and other visual artists, dancers, and meditation specialists into our halls, public spaces, and patient rooms. The program emphasized the personal side of the doctor–patient equation, and a few times I even brought my guitar and played in workshops. I wasn't entirely comfortable with that, even within the context of the arts program. I loved doing it, but I worried I might look less professional—less like a doctor—if I let my guard down so completely within the hospital's walls. After all, I was still just a fellow, still trying to prove myself in an incredibly rigorous academic program, and still losing my lunch on a regular basis when one of the tougher professors criticized my work. I was also the only fellow with a D.O. after my name instead of an M.D., and I wanted to represent osteopathic training the best I could.

I began to suspect my insecurities in that area were unfounded around the time Nancy sponsored a juried art show and contest for patients and staff. I brought in my "masterpiece"—a painting I'd done in college by intently studying my reflection in the mirror and then dabbing oil paints on the canvas with my hands. It hung in the main lobby of the cancer center for a few weeks and eventually won first prize.

I spotted Dr. Jekyll in the hall one afternoon and pivoted, hoping to escape his notice.

I was too slow. He called out my name, and I turned to face him for whatever abuse was coming.

"You've really got something there," he said.

"Sir?"

"That *painting*. It's great." Then he patted my shoulder and continued down the hall.

Wait. What? A compliment from the man who routinely shredded me in front of my professors and peers? *Eisenberg! Amateur!* He liked my painting. He had touched me. Had he smiled? What the hell was happening?

The experiment of the arts and humanities program took on new depth for me that day. It had broken down the one barrier I'd never dreamed could be dismantled. Jekyll acknowledged me as a human with feelings and talent. I started to think he might be a man and not a monster.

The benefits of the arts program were palpable all over the hospital. Patients, families, doctors, nurses, aides, and administrators often participated together. Sharing music or a dance recital, an art contest or a writing exercise, broke through the formalities of our respective roles and helped us simply connect. It was personal, and that carried over into exam rooms and office meetings and surgical suites, making us more comfortable with one another and fostering genuine shared interests and empathy.

Everything about the program felt right to me. Sometimes I wondered if I should hand out copies of Bocelli's *Sogno,* or musical instruments, or Three Stooges videos, or fresh notebooks begging to be filled one day at a time. Instead I tried to ask each patient—and still do—*What's your favorite song? Favorite color? What movie makes you laugh? What book makes you cry? What fairy tale did you most love to read to your children?*

And then we would compare notes and get to know one another. Those first appointments are likely, hopefully, the beginning of long relationships. We will be co-conspirators against cancer. The promises are implicit in the connection: *I will be your ally if you will be my patient. When you need me, I will take the lead. When you ask, I will follow yours. If we can trust each other, talk to each other, laugh and cry together, we'll be a powerful team.*

None of us wants to face cancer, but at some point most of us will. It may be our own, or that of someone we love, but very few walk through this life unscathed. Given that reality, shouldn't doctors and patients find our way to true partnerships? And isn't it better for everyone if those partnerships encompass things we love instead of just the one thing we all hate?

At this writing it's been 20 years since Ken and I sang "What a Wonderful World" during his bone marrow extraction, and I've sung and danced and joked and written and painted and done deep breathing with thousands of patients. When I look back, it's easy to see how often those moments opened up lines of communication that ultimately contributed to better care, more comfort, and greater healing than would have been possible if they'd remained closed. Those relationships are my masterpieces, the collaborations that make me proud.

So how do you take the cancer center's arts and humanities program and these relationships that aren't always easy to come by and put them to use in your own fight against disease? Start by picking up a pen. If you are fighting cancer (or any other disease), I encourage you to write down how you're feeling, what makes you mad, and what would make you feel better. Write down your questions, your symptoms, your fears, and your hopes. Write down how much you effing hate your caustic chemo or your itchy wig or hearing people say *Hang in there*, as if there were a lot of viable alternatives.

Use your writing to figure out what you want to say to your doctor and family and friends. Then take it a step further and write a letter. It can be to anyone—your future self, your grandmother in heaven, your mother in Sacramento, your son who's away at college, your oncologist. Maybe there's someone you want to thank, or maybe someone you want to forgive. Maybe you want to share a memory or ask for a favor or just describe the beautiful blooming tree outside your window. The important thing is to express yourself. It is the first step toward being heard.

CHAPTER 5

THIS TOO WILL PASS

One thing.
The one thing you control is your response.
Your response to what happens.
That's it.

— *DAILY DOSE*, OCTOBER 14, 2020

I was learning more every day about how to take care of my patients. I could design treatments and medicate side effects with increasing confidence. But I was having a hard time figuring out how to interact with and somehow comfort patients overwhelmed by the emotional toll of illness and treatment. There was little in the curriculum to address the fact that patients were showing up shocked, depressed, or seething with anger. My professors handled this side of care with widely varying personal styles. Some would take extra time to hear out each patient's concerns, acknowledging his or her feelings and offering empathy. Some would offer prescriptions for antidepressants or referrals to counselors or group therapy. Some would steer dialogue away from personal issues as quickly as they arose, turning businesslike to discourage patients from getting emotional.

As someone who was spending countless hours at home trying to work through my own pain at just witnessing what my patients and their families were going through, I knew I could never shut down a patient who needed to talk or weep or rage to try to protect my schedule or my emotions. But I didn't know what I had to offer them besides a sympathetic ear.

One of my favorite songwriters during my time at Georgetown (and still) was an artist named Peter Himmelman. I'd seen him play a couple times in Philadelphia and been fascinated by and envious of his authentic, imaginative, eloquent lyrics. I bet I played his albums a thousand times, so it's no wonder that many of his lyrics were part of the soundtrack of my years in fellowship. I often heard his song "This Too Will Pass" in my head as I went from one patient room to the next, and I occasionally caught myself singing it aloud in the hallway. Depending on how things were going, sometimes I put my emphasis on his observation that some days seem like they'll drag on forever, and others on the line proclaiming things will get better.

It is the privilege and the burden of an oncologist to be in the room with patients at some of the most significant, devastating, and elating moments of their lives. There's an intimacy to it that nothing in training prepares you for. When you say the words that cause a grown person to weep or moan, shake with anger, shriek with joy, or spontaneously begin to pray, you are a part of something, and yet outside of it. You aspire to be a healer, but you must also be a good messenger, and a good listener.

♡

As a fellow it was my job to go through each new patient's medical records, then conduct a visit to get a history and all the other pertinent information, and finally present the case to the attending physician. One of the first patients I managed on my own was a young woman who had her two small children with her. Tracy had been diagnosed with stage IV breast cancer and her condition was ultimately incurable. But she had survived her chemo and was stronger for having done it. In a million years I could never get used to telling young women, young mothers, that they have this cancer and that it is a hard one to treat. Even then I knew being able to say *You're in remission* was the best I could dare to hope for.

But when I said it, Tracy broke down, burying her face in her hands. I asked what was going on, and she said she wasn't able to sleep or enjoy her time with her family. She couldn't celebrate the success of the chemo. She was so afraid of her cancer coming back that it was all she could think about.

She said she couldn't even look at her beautiful children without thinking that she might leave them without a mother, without wondering if they would remember her.

I asked questions I'd heard other oncologists ask: *Do you have anyone you can talk to about this? Are you taking any medications for anxiety? How much exercise are you getting?*

At the exercise question, Tracy turned her head toward her son and daughter, who were playing in the corner, and didn't answer. I could feel that I was failing her. Yes, exercise is a critical tool in combatting anxiety; but no, that wasn't what she needed from me in the moment.

I wheeled my stool closer to her chair, so we were knee to knee, and hoped the right words would come to me. "Tracy, you are always going to worry about cancer. That's a normal, natural response to what you've been through. Everyone who's been through this is afraid."

Tracy nodded and wiped away tears as I tried to think of anything I could possibly say that might help her. "You're doing everything in your power to control the disease, and you're doing an amazing job," I said. "Look at you—so strong after chemotherapy. And your new scans are beautiful. Completely clear."

"I know," she said, her voice shaky. "I know, but I can't let it go—and I am draining myself and my husband, my sisters, and my mother, just everyone in my life right now." Again, her gaze went to her children, and mine followed. They were sitting side by side, scribbling on facing pages of a coloring book.

I wanted to scream at the tragic irony of Tracy spending any of her precious time with them obsessing about her cancer. Instead I replayed her words in my head and fixated on *let it go.*

This too will pass.

I thought about how I'd been coping, about everything I'd learned about meditation in college and since, and decided that maybe I could help her pivot her focus from the tenuous future to the possible present.

"I can't tell you if or when your cancer will come back," I said. "But I think right now the trick is that you have to accept your pain before you can let it go. You can't just push it away without acknowledging it. You have to let it in, then let it go."

Face them. Embrace them. Replace them.

That was the first time I ever taught a patient how to meditate in an exam room. Tracy and I walked through the simple steps of meditation using a mantra I learned from Deepak Chopra. We sat calmly, breathing deeply, repeating the mantra: *Soooo. Hummm.* I told her that her mind was going to try to race back to where she'd just come from, and she could acknowledge her fears and say, "Okay. Thank you," and get back to her mantra. We talked about how she was far more than the sum of her fearful thoughts, more than her disease. I told her it was within her power to both accept those burdens and set them aside.

After a few minutes of meditation, Tracy said, "That's the closest thing to peace I've felt in months." She agreed to keep it up, practicing it like she'd take an essential medication, twice a day, every day.

Watching her bundle her kids into their coats and scarves to leave, I was struck by how much I still had to learn. This wasn't in the curriculum, but Tracy's fears were as disruptive and painful as any physical symptom. I would have given anything to be able to offer her a cure, but all I had for her that day was a coping mechanism.

♡

Just as I saw patients who were overwhelmed with fear, I saw others who faced their cancer with another emotion: fury. Some were prepared to go to any lengths to strike back at their disease. One of these was a tall middle-aged woman named Sylvia who had metastatic ovarian cancer. She was one of the most determined fighters I'd ever seen. She was in Georgetown's ICU when we first met, with more tubes keeping her alive than seemed possible. She had one to drain fluid from her belly, which had been swollen and tight as a drum without it. She had one that went through her nostril to her stomach so we could feed her, one to drain her bowels, another to drain her kidneys. She somehow managed to walk with all of it, and she was *constantly* asking for yet another treatment, no matter how experimental or aggressive. There was a new chemo regimen in clinical trial for ovarian patients, and she wanted it. She was already standing at the ragged edge of death, but her will to live was fierce. What Sylvia was asking for in her condition was like volunteering to stand in front of a firing squad—except she was doing it to live, not to die. Her fighting spirit was infectious, and I found that I seemed to carry it with me after each visit with her, meting it out in bursts of positivity and determination to each patient I saw afterward.

Patients like Sylvia were the reason that, despite the grueling hours and the outcomes of some of our cases, there were times when we residents were privy to glimmers of exquisite promise—signs of payoffs for the studies and the research and the Sylvias who fearlessly put themselves forward to test new treatments.

A pill called Gleevec was the first biologic treatment on my radar—used against a type of blood cancer called chronic myelogenous leukemia (CML). There was a time when a diagnosis of CML was essentially a death sentence. In the 1960s researchers tied the rare cancer to a genetic abnormality they named the Philadelphia chromosome. Thirty years later, and with a better understanding of how the genetic mutation created the cancer, another research team postulated that if they could find a drug that would singularly root out cells caused by this abnormality, they could cure the disease.

Gleevec was that drug. One of the first medical marvels I ever saw was a patient who came to the hospital in dire shape and responded to Gleevec almost immediately. One day he was indisputably dying; the next he was sitting up in his bed, playing cards with his brother. The pill targeted only the cancer-causing cells, so it spared patients the harshest side effects of chemotherapy. It could be taken long term, and in the years that followed, studies found it was built to last. The five-year survival rate skyrocketed, and just like that, CML was a largely treatable disease.

Gleevec was a silver bullet. It was also a harbinger of things to come, of treatments that pinpoint specific kinds of cells and destroy or block them. This was the dawn of targeted treatment, the possibilities of which we are still exploring and expanding day by day and year by year.

CHAPTER 6

BEAUTIFUL DAY

In the middle of the night
I remember
My oldest friends, my grandparents
My parents, my sister
Aunts, uncles, cousins, nieces, nephews
Family
I make sure my wife and kids are tucked in
I remember what matters

— *DAILY DOSE*, APRIL 11, 2020

Most of us have lived with cancer in one form or another—because it has touched our own health or that of someone we love. For me it was both grandmothers. My aunt. My father's favorite cousin. And nearly two decades ago, while I was still finding my way as an oncology fellow, it was my teenage sister-in-law.

More than any other, hers was the case that made me realize that all of us who go through this experience are one big, complicated, chaotic family. Like any family, we need each other, and we need to love each other.

In December of 2000, as I was driving to work at the Lombardi Center, my stereo blaring U2's new hit *Beautiful Day*, I got an urgent phone call from my mother-in-law. My wife Julie's 15-year-old sister was sick. Brittany had woken early that morning with her heart racing, her head pounding, and her vision blurred. Within minutes she'd passed out. Something was seriously wrong. At the local emergency room, there was no quick diagnosis, but Brittany was not improving, and my mother-in-law, Nancy, refused to leave without some explanation. By the time she called me, someone had taken a closer look at Brittany's blood cells. The ER doctor believed the culprit could be leukemia. Did the family have an oncologist, he asked, or would they like to be referred to the one on duty at the hospital?

I was stunned to get the call. I'd been concerned about Brittany's health ever since she'd had a case of shingles—something children rarely get—but I hadn't seen this coming. Since I was working in a top cancer center, the first step was getting Brittany released to Georgetown. Nancy didn't hesitate. As soon as they were on their way, I went searching for Dr. Aziza Shad, a pediatric leukemia specialist whose work I respected and admired. Dr. Shad agreed to accept Brittany as her patient.

That night Julie told me that during the transfer between hospitals, Brittany was the sickest she had ever seen anyone in her life. "She was barely with us," she said.

A round of tests that included a bone marrow sample revealed that Brittany was suffering from full-blown acute myelogenous leukemia (AML), an aggressive blood cancer that's usually found in older adults. It starts when a single cell's DNA mutates in the bone marrow, and it escalates as that cell divides into two, and those into four, and so on, with the number of unhealthy cells growing exponentially. Unlike most cancers, which take the form of a growing mass, leukemia cells invade the patient's bloodstream and make their way throughout the body.

The prognosis was dismal. At the time most kids Brittany's age with AML did not survive it. Her life and those of my in-laws changed completely that day as they put their careers on hold and narrowed their focus to the hospital and their young daughter. Julie was pregnant with our first child, and she and I huddled together in disbelief. I pictured the baby we were going to have in a few months, appalled at how vulnerable he or she was going to be in the world. I said a prayer for my beloved in-laws, who'd immediately adopted safety protocols to protect Brittany's fragile immune system and staked out a corner of her reverse-ventilation room at the hospital with little more than a duffle bag and a cot. And as I thought of the patients I was seeing every day in my leukemia rotation, I was struck with a new level of understanding of what they were facing, of just how terrifying a river of disease flowing in your own blood can be. This was not something that could be cut away. It would take a different and more total kind of intervention.

I met with Dr. Shad on the family's behalf and recognized both the hope and the danger of the experimental treatment regimen she proposed. Brittany would have been diagnosed with AML if 20 out of every 100 white blood cells in her marrow were leukemic (aka blast cells). Her levels were more than three times that threshold. Her life was in immediate peril, and the only chance Dr. Shad saw to save her was to go after the white blood cells with such a powerful chemotherapy agent that they'd be wiped out—the healthy ones along with the blasts.

The family put their trust entirely in me; I put mine in Dr. Shad; and the plan was set in motion.

During what felt like the coldest, darkest winter of our lives, Brittany underwent multiple in-patient rounds of extremely aggressive chemo. She struggled to survive her treatment. There were many times when it seemed that she would not make it, that she was too weak to recover. We had known the risks and known that without the treatment she wouldn't have a chance. It was a cruel choice for everyone who loved her—subject her to the harshest regimen imaginable, or give up.

Every day I'd visit between rounds, slipping into Brittany's room to watch a few minutes of her favorite movie or tell her a joke or just see how she looked, which was very small and pale. I always wore a mask over my face and came with my hands practically dripping with Purell to keep from bringing any trace of contaminant in contact with her fragile system. When I brought my guitar in for the arts and humanities program, I stopped by to play for Brittany too. I'd wipe it down in the hall to clear off any germs, then sing through my surgical mask. "Beauty and the Beast" was a favorite, so I'd lead with its theme, crooning, *"Tale as old as time . . ."*

The two of us had always bonded over our shared love of musicals, singing out lyrics and quoting lines to each other, but most days during treatment she was too weak to sing along.

When Brittany lost her hair and developed lesions and painful inflammation in her digestive tract, I started calling her Brittany-Belle, and reminded her every day that she was strong and beautiful. Her mom and dad and Julie took turns staying with her, never wanting her to feel alone. She was surrounded by love and support.

After four months in the hospital, Brittany was sent home to wait, to see if her bone marrow—completely destroyed by the chemo—could grow back healthy. I explained it to her in terms she could understand by talking about bone marrow as real estate.

"You had these wild, bad cells that moved in," I said, "and they were throwing crazy parties and trashing the place. They had to go. Now that they're out, your regular cells—the good neighbors—can move back in and help you get back to normal."

But Brittany's bone marrow was a ghost town. For months after completion of her chemo, no one moved back in. Every day of the wait she was so weak and vulnerable that any germ, any virus, any kind of infection could have killed her. Nurses came to the house to draw her blood and she trekked back and forth to the hospital for bone marrow biopsies and red blood cell and platelet transfusions to keep her alive. My in-laws and Julie and I watched and worried, and I fumed over the idea that her research protocol—the one I encouraged the family to accept—had worked so well that it might ultimately kill her.

Two hundred days passed—the longest stretch the hospital had ever seen during which a patient had zero blood counts.

Julie's pregnancy progressed. I wrestled with the daily strain of oncology. And Brittany's health was always at the forefront of our thoughts.

Late in the spring, we got our first miracle. Brittany—gaunt, pale, jaundiced, and by then 16 years old—began to heal. Feeling the love around her, the unconditional devotion of her parents and her sister and me, she grabbed onto that little bit of hope and something shifted in her. Her bone marrow counts slowly started to rise. Dr. Shad and I huddled again, this time in the understanding that the aggressive protocol that nearly killed Brittany had in fact saved her—completely wiping out her cancer and allowing her body, in its own time, to renew. She was going to be a survivor.

In the summer we were given a second miracle. Our baby girl, Kaiya, was born. Brittany was still recovering, and as I watched her cradle Kaiya, I felt that no matter what heartbreak oncology could throw at me, moments like that, shining with hope and redemption and possibility, would carry me through. I felt willing to accept it all—burdens and blessings—for as long as I could absorb the raw emotions that come part and parcel with the work. I hoped it would be a long, long while.

That afternoon I told Brittany how incredibly happy I was that she had gotten a second chance. I put my arm around her and gave her the same advice my dad had given me: *Don't ever take your life for granted.*

"You and I," I told her, "we're the lucky ones."

♡

Helping to treat and console a member of my family brought all the work I'd been doing in the oncology department into sharp focus. I had seen for months how critical it was to keep the thread between Brittany and the family taut and energized and positive. I had felt the desperation to do something, anything, to help.

For three years learning about oncology had shaped my life and experience every single day, determining how I spent my waking hours, if and when I slept, how I felt about myself and the world. But going through Brittany's illness alongside her, feeling the anguish and hopes of illness and treatment as a member of my family, a child, endured them, added an emotional depth to the experience that was almost too much to take. Rather than push me away from the field, it drew me closer. As we moved on from Brittany's illness, I promised myself I'd never forget just how total the cancer experience is for the family. If I was going to be the kind of doctor I aspired to be, I'd have to find a way to treat each family like my family, to care enough that they could feel it.

Ever since those days of my fellowship, when I meet a new patient, I envision that person as part of my own extended family. Sometimes I tell them: *I'm going to treat you like I would treat my sister, my mother, my father, my brother.* Sometimes it goes unsaid. But that sense that the best possible cancer care comes from a far deeper connection than just a doctor–patient dynamic has never left me since the days when Brittany endured, then survived, her cancer and its treatment.

I see that same loving attitude being fostered every day by the other doctors in my practice, by nurses and office staff, by patients and families who share small kindnesses with each other in the treatment room, and by volunteers who call to ask what they can do. I see veteran patients offering advice and encouragement to the newly diagnosed, and sometimes the mom of one patient rubbing the back or patting the hand of another. Each of us whose lives have been touched by cancer is part of this giant family, and we owe it to one another to interact with kindness and empathy.

If you are struggling, reach out to a member of your family or ask your oncologist to recommend someone who can encourage you. If you are feeling strong, if you are cured, remember your brothers and sisters, uncles and aunts, grandparents and cousins who are still in the fight. Look on one another with kindness. Uncle Manny, my beloved professor at PCOM, was a huge proponent of the *watch one, do one, teach one* philosophy. "If you learn well," he told us, "the time will come when it falls to you to keep the faith." I know he was talking about us as medical students, but I like to think his advice—like all his good guidance—applies to me in and out of my white coat, and that his words of wisdom are easily applied to everyone.

CHAPTER 7

STUCK IN A MOMENT

You see darkness.
And it's okay.
Go into your cave and embrace it.
Shut down.
Refuel.
Revitalize your heart.
And it's okay.

— *Daily Dose*, July 25, 2019

One key step we can all take—especially when we're going through hard times—is choosing to share our burden with people we care about who care back. Personally, I had to learn this lesson on the business side of oncology before I could truly appreciate its significance in terms of therapeutic value.

At the end of my fellowship, I accepted an offer to join a private oncology practice in San Diego. I went to California bursting with hope—about the kind of oncologist I was going to be, the kind of practice I'd be working in, the way I was going to change lives. I wish I could say that's exactly how things came together, but it wasn't long at all before I stumbled, caught out by the realization that life in private practice was nothing like I'd imagined it would be. In fact, not a single minute of my decade of med school, internship, and fellowship prepared me for operating within the business model to which my new colleagues were beholden. Insiders call it the *eat what you kill* model—a common way of doing business for private law and medical practices. In theory this system with a brutal name offers a logical approach to running a group office: each doctor bills for and keeps compensation from his or her own patient encounters, minus shared office expenses. In practice, however, this method can reflect all the negative connotations the name implies—medical professionals preying on certain victims because they're "hungry" rather than because of patient need, doctors "poaching" patients from office mates and other practices, "lions" of the practice's pride demanding a piece of everyone else's take. The end result was as bad as you can imagine—a bunch of highly trained medical professionals who wanted to be focused first and foremost on their roles as healers seemingly trapped in an environment with all the drama and dysfunction of a Kardashian episode.

The effects were toxic. The new office even had an accountant who was constantly doing the math that would determine if we'd met our quotas and earned our salaries for the month or if we were *negative*—a word he'd say in a way that implied every last thing about you was negative, not just your account.

I was expected to focus on the business of oncology at least as much as the practice of it, and this was new to me. Until I got to San Diego, I'd been a student of one kind or another, and my role had always been to simply treat whoever showed up. This seemed like the most obvious way to run any medical office, but instead I was under mounting pressure to build a practice, and to do it by being seen, by endearing myself to hospitals and primary care practices, and even by outpacing my partners. Under this model, the more patients I saw every day, the more successful I'd supposedly be—an assumption that flew in the face of my habit of taking as much time as each patient needed. An oncology practice is a small business, but it's not one you can build or effectively measure in terms of productivity and profitability. The work demands a better measure than that.

I was a young, idealistic doctor who wanted to get to know my patients, to weigh every treatment's benefits against its dangers, to integrate things like meditation and music and nutrition and exercise into my practice (none of which had any measurable value in the profit-first business model). More than anything, I wanted to be a healer, a consoler, a bringer of hope—and I was discovering that the world I'd chosen expected—demanded—something entirely different.

The immediate consequence of these new, noxious priorities was that I didn't have enough time for my patients or for my family. My guitar—forget about it. It sat in a corner, gathering dust. I felt like a naive, foolish kid who'd been playing doctor for years, only to discover that the real world was nothing like his childish game of hospital.

♡

It was during this frustrating, challenging time that I first met Lydia. A senior member of the practice dropped a file on my desk, saying that the patient was difficult but the case would help me build my billing. Per her record, Lydia was a 50-year-old breast cancer patient who was noncompliant in almost every way. Sometimes she didn't show up for appointments—even for carefully timed chemo treatments. Sometimes she snapped at the nurses. Sometimes she raised her voice in the hushed quiet of the waiting room, and sometimes she swore a blue streak when she got frustrated.

Lydia had shown signs of mental instability from the beginning of her relationship with the practice, and she always came alone.

The most notable medical matter in Lydia's file, though, was that she had weathered one terrible side effect after another during her treatment, and that she'd suffered heart damage as a result of her chemo regimen. Sometimes a patient's heart can't take the treatment—because of an undiagnosed preexisting condition or because the dose that's required to destroy the cancer is more than the organ can tolerate. This is a calculation every oncologist must make before offering chemotherapy. The probability of cancer survival typically outweighs the small chance of serious complications, and that was Lydia's case. Without treatment there was no question she would not have survived.

Understandably, there was no medical explanation that made Lydia feel any less angry about her condition. Why would it? She had made a leap of faith and followed a protocol that had taken more away from her than the cancer alone. With no one else to blame, she directed her frustration at her medical team.

I came into our first appointment together eager to smooth out the prickly relationship Lydia had come to have with everyone in the office.

She wasn't happy to see me.

"And *who* are *you?*" she demanded when I walked into the exam room. Her skin had an ashy pall and her breathing was labored. I knew she was 50, but she appeared at least 10 years older. She looked me over, her eyes searching my face, waiting for an answer.

I told her I was going to start overseeing her care and that I wanted to know how she was feeling so I could figure out how I could help her.

"How I feel is *sick*," she snapped. "Sick all the time, and tired."

"Okay," I answered. "Let's see what we can do about that. Tell me more about where and when and how you feel sick."

As we explored her symptoms, I asked more questions: *Is it your stomach? Do you have headaches? Are there times of the day when it is worse than others? How much water are you drinking? What's your diet like? Are you constipated? How often are you taking your as-needed medications? Are they helping? Have you ever taken an antidepressant?*

By the end of our first round of this joyless version of 20 questions, I had a better sense of how Lydia was feeling and what measures I might be able to offer to help her.

In the months that followed, we developed a complicated but functional relationship. She certainly didn't like me, but I thought maybe she could tell I was committed to helping her. Each time I tried to connect on a deeper level, though, she shut me down. When I asked if she had anyone to take a walk with her, to take her shopping, or to help her better manage her regimen of medications, she clapped back, hard.

"I don't need any more damn help," she said. She didn't want to meet a patient advocate, didn't want the number for the local support group, didn't want to see me if she could help it.

It was so clear that Lydia blamed the practice for her deteriorating condition that I reread her file a dozen times or more, trying to pinpoint the exact moments when things went wrong and if there was any point in her care when we'd failed her. Each review seemed to retell the same story—a string of procedures and appointments that had gone badly. Each of them could have happened to anyone, but they had all happened to this one lonely, unstable, insecure woman who never seemed to catch a break.

The ability to connect with patients had been my strength ever since med school, but this was someone who didn't want connection. Each time I asked a question, she stonewalled and scowled.

It might sound like this was my problem—just an insecure guy upset because a lady didn't like him. But it was bigger than that. I was her doctor, and if she didn't have trust in me, I could only do half my job. There is both art and science to practicing medicine. At that moment in Lydia's life, the science was up to date. She had been diagnosed, treated, and prescribed an estrogen-blocking medication to discourage cancer recurrence. I had scavenged as much information as possible about the ongoing symptoms she was experiencing and made appropriate medical recommendations. But the art of the matter was in whether I'd conveyed their importance sufficiently and whether we'd built enough trust for Lydia to choose to follow through.

For at least a century, scientists have studied the dynamics of the doctor–patient relationship (so much so that it has an acronym: DPR), and what those studies find, time and again and in one form or another, is that the relationship is an independent factor in patient compliance with doctors' instructions. Sometimes it's the only factor we can pin down. I had come to medicine with a knack and a passion for building relationships and trust—I hadn't needed to study how to do that. Sadly, this patient, who was the first to truly and deliberately wall herself off from me and from everyone else in the practice, was one who could suffer significant consequences if she skipped pills or otherwise neglected her care.

♡

Despite the fact that I was doing good work with other patients and managing to stay on the positive side of the accountant's ledgers, it felt to me like Lydia's case went hand in hand with my frustrations with the system in which I felt trapped. It took a turn for the worse the first time she missed an appointment with me. For months I'd seen her not just at her every-12-weeks checkup, but also frequently in between. Sometimes she'd call and make an appointment; more often, despite the fact that she professed not to want to see me, she'd simply show up and wait. After the appointment she missed, the office called and left a message with a rescheduled time, but she didn't show up for that appointment either. I tried to call her myself but got no answer. Weeks passed and I knew she must be out of medication to mitigate the side effects she'd been living with. And she was likely also out of tamoxifen, the hormone-inhibiting treatment that lowered her chances of a recurrence. She was in the wind, and I was so stressed out by her case and the pressures of the job and the infighting among the members of my team that instead of sleeping at night, I focused on this lost patient. I imagined her somewhere out in the city, alone and sick and angry.

During these months my own health began to suffer. The asthma I'd had as a child resurfaced, and I had to get my first new inhaler in a decade. I was diagnosed with optical migraines that caused not just excruciating pain but also temporary blindness. I developed insomnia and felt an ever-worsening anxiety. I had symptoms of fibromyalgia— muscle and joint pain and a sluggishness I couldn't shake. I made an appointment to see a rheumatologist, who ran a few tests and got straight to the point.

"You're not sick, Steven," he said emphatically. "You need to deal with whatever is causing all of this stress."

Maybe it was an early midlife crisis, a reality check on my best intentions, or a test of faith, but I was losing my hope during this adjustment to private practice.

Every day in the office, I tried to get my groove back. Every night at home, I tried to shake off the weight of the day and be present for my family. I felt frustration and guilt and regret—as if Lydia's chemotherapy was somehow responsible not just for her heart condition, but also for this whole angry, unhappy phase of her life.

♡

I don't know what ultimately happened to Lydia. I still think of her often and pray she is healthy and well. What happened to me, though, was that I met another doctor who was willing to help me sort through my jumble of guilt and frustration and make some sense of it.

Within the structure of a hospital or medical practice, team members often assemble a tumor board of oncology experts who can consult together about complex cases. I was invited to serve on this board at a hospital where I saw patients, and that's where I met Dr. Victor Kovner. He was 30 or more years older than I, and his area of specialization was hospice care. It takes a dedicated and selfless soul to embrace the work of providing palliative care, of helping ease patients out of this life and on to the next, and I instantly respected Victor for his choice. I instantly liked him too, when he shook my hand and smiled broadly and welcomed me to the "club." Soon we were meeting for lunch and talking about what we could do to improve the hospital's care. The answer that bubbled up tapped directly into what was going on in my own life. Victor wanted to create a program that would encourage doctors and nurses to express their grief, frustrations, and struggles with patient care in a safe environment. And he generously, thoughtfully listened when a discussion about this project prompted me to share the guilt and angst I was feeling about Lydia—whose case I described while being careful to protect her privacy. I referred to her as "the heart lady," and Victor nodded in understanding.

Victor reminded me that when I chose oncology, I knew my career would be touched by loss—not just once in a while, but continually. We talked about how one of the only positive aspects of a cancer diagnosis is the way it opens doors for all kinds of second chances—to live, to love, to make authentic choices outside the bounds of the social pressures that seem to fall away when you are living with the possibility of dying.

He said that in his experience, there are always patients who are too wounded or grief-stricken or frustrated or angry to embrace any of it, and that is always their right.

"You've done everything you can do for your heart lady," he said. "She is a survivor. It's time to let her go."

♡

One of the things we all—patients, caregivers, families—have to discover in our own time about cancer and its treatment is that our experience of it is about far more than just winning and losing against the disease. It's about more than the pain and the side effects and the exhaustion of going through treatment. It is often a turning point in our lives on many more planes than just the medical. I see patients every day who are awake to life in ways they haven't been in years, even decades. I see families who are healing and lost love being found. I see people who are funny, who are angry, who are praying, who are making amends or offering forgiveness.

I had patients who were doing better and patients who were doing worse, but it was Lydia's case that haunted me. Looking back I realize the root of this, the reason it was so impossible to accept, was her almost total sense of abandonment, her hopelessness. She shut herself off from the world, and to this day she remains one of the few patients I feel

I failed because I couldn't find a way to help her. Worse, I knew she didn't have anyone else.

At the time there was no lesson in it for me—just despair. But today I think of Lydia often as I encourage families to pull together, to forgive and mend. I think of her when I spend extra time and energy making sure patients who live alone have the support they need at home. I think of her when I encourage patients to express whatever emotions they are feeling, no matter what, in the hopes that they can get to a point of peace. That objective is the same whether you're on your way to a cure or on your way to a terminal diagnosis. I believe that every human being alive has a heart longing for a moment of peace. A cancer diagnosis can reveal a shortcut to it, but it can also open a trapdoor that drops you down and away.

In truth, I've been an oncologist long enough now to know that fear, confusion, and hopelessness can take over very quickly—like a few seconds after bad news. They are the trapdoor—away from healing, away from empowerment, away from peace. The trick to avoiding that trapdoor is remembering that *how* you are doing is correlated with *what* you are doing. Tiny actions lead to feeling a tiny bit better, a tiny bit closer to where you want to be. So instead of shutting down, meet one of your most basic obligations, and then another. Eat something healthy; walk when you can; take your medicine; listen to your favorite song; keep your appointments; talk with your family; call your friend; tell someone you love them; watch a funny movie or reread that book you love. Do the things you must and do the things you love—that's the oncology patient's equivalent to putting one foot in front of the other, moving away from that chasm of hopelessness a little at a time. Inching closer to peace.

CHAPTER 8

LET IT BE

We have great power.
The power to accept life just as it is,
And just as it isn't.

— *DAILY DOSE*, NOVEMBER 18, 2017

While I was trying to push through my early career crisis and also prioritize my young family at home, I was failing to follow my doctor's advice. I was no closer to resolving my stress issues than I'd been in months.

In what felt like the final insult from my body, my skin started to itch. At first it was just a little here and there, but it got worse, resulting in little red bumps that made me look like I'd lost a fight with a nest of spiders. I chalked it up to a messed-up immune system. I was off my game on so many levels—of course my skin would want in on the revolt.

I added steroid and anti-itch creams to my long list of medical interventions. But one afternoon as I raked my fingernails across my chest, they snagged on something different, a raised bump on my left pec, almost directly over my heart. Touching it made it itchier, and for a few days it became the main focus in my rotating cast of ailments.

Skin bumps come and go, and mine fell into step with my diminishing weight, asthma, headaches, and the stomachaches that plagued me at night. I knew something had to change, but I wasn't sure how to swing the tide as my health issues steadily beat me down.

The irony wasn't lost on me that these stress-related health problems—things I could theoretically control—were chipping away at how much energy and focus I had for my patients. I strove to give 100 percent in every exam room, but I had a sense that perhaps I was falling short.

Weeks after I first noticed the bump on my chest, I caught sight of it in the mirror and stared. It was round and hard and white, like a tiny pearl. It felt more than skin deep, as if it was rooted in my chest wall. This was not a bump to ignore.

I called a dermatologist friend, and she said (and I quote because this is sound advice), "Anything that doesn't go away in a month, you need to get your butt to a doctor." She took a shave biopsy, and when she called with the results, she didn't mince words.

"It's a basal cell carcinoma, and it needs to be excised immediately."

Of course it was. I was in such a bad place I felt like I deserved it, like maybe I'd even brought it on. Like it was a fitting punishment for a miserable oncologist who couldn't get his shit together. Intellectually I knew better than to think any of that, but my emotions were all over the place, running wild with crazy ideas about things that were essentially impossible.

A week later I was sitting in an office surgical suite, humming the Beatles' "Let It Be," waiting for the excision to get underway. Paul McCartney, I remembered reading somewhere, lost his mother to cancer when he was just a teenager. She is the Mother Mary in the song. The song had resonated with me all my life—as a songwriter, a musician, a Beatles fan, a mama's boy, and a parent. That day I couldn't get it out of my head.

Dr. Chen used a Sharpie pen to mark the site on my chest. The shape of it looked like a pair of lips, wider than tall, rounded in the middle. I knew she'd need to achieve five millimeters of clear margin on all sides, but I hadn't thought much about the depth of the lesion—that it would require her to excise deep below the skin.

She scrubbed the area and administered a lidocaine injection to numb it. Over the next hour, she painstakingly excised the pearly lump and the tissue around it, then sewed the wound closed with several stitches. While she worked I watched her eyes peering over her surgical mask. The moment swept me back nearly 20 years to the hours I'd spent watching Dr. Kodsi's face as he reconstructed the damage from my bike-wreck injuries. Dr. Chen offered steady commentary on what she was doing and how it was going, not bothering to pare down the medical jargon because we both knew it well. I freely admit, though, that for that hour I felt as much like I was my 13-year-old injured self again as I did like a physician with years of specialized training.

Driving home, I thought about my patients and the surgeries so many of them had endured. Lumpectomies and mastectomies, colectomies and hysterectomies, excisions from their livers and lungs and kidneys. My operation was small by comparison—an hour in a sterile office, no IV sedation or breathing tube or hospital stay required—but it made me feel closer to the women and men I was treating and their experience. It also forced me to think about how damn lucky I was. I knew as well as anyone alive how quickly and cruelly one little sign that something is wrong in the body can be the beginning of an avalanche of tests, diagnoses, and treatments. In relative terms my excision was a story with a happy ending: Cancer found. Removed completely. The end.

My procedure left me with a scar a couple inches wide almost directly over my heart, a physical, forever reminder of a time in my life when I was struggling to be the doctor and the man I aspired to be.

♡

When I first moved to San Diego, I was looking for new possibilities, and I'd imagined being in the sun and near the ocean would help ease the inevitable stress of oncology practice. In the beginning I often drove out to the beach to watch the sun set over the ocean—nature's magic trick at the end of each day. But months passed and I stopped going toward or thinking about sunsets, because I was too wrapped up in my anxiety and my growing list of ailments and distractions.

There were others, though, who had come to the California coast and not lost sight of its unique beauty. High in the hills around the city and its suburbs, dozens of monasteries representing a wide range of faiths and cultures make the most of the scenic, sheltered setting—using it as a place to worship, meditate, teach, and sometimes to find refuge from persecution elsewhere.

My excision scar was still healing when a patient came down from one of these mountain sanctuaries and into my office. His unique history and temperament would offer me some needed perspective.

I happened to be in the waiting room when the monk arrived. He was quintessential, everything I imagined a monk to be, from his smooth shaved head to his long red and yellow robes to the wire-rimmed glasses resting over kind, knowing eyes. He had a slight build, maybe five-foot-three or four, and he weighed no more than 130 pounds, but his presence filled the room. I instinctively bowed a little bit when I saw him.

I've always been fascinated by religion—not just the Jewish faith I was raised in, but all of them. In my years of practice and witnessing the ways faith inspires and strengthens families in their most difficult times, that interest has only intensified. The arrival of a Tibetan Buddhist monk in my waiting room felt like a moment I'd been waiting for, and it challenged and humbled me to be a physician worthy of providing his care.

The monk spoke softly and evenly in a language in which I couldn't recognize a single syllable. The translator who'd accompanied him conveyed his words to me. They explained that he'd developed a persistent cough and that after some time he'd seen an internal medicine doctor and had been referred for a chest X-ray. When the X-ray came back with a suspicious but unidentifiable shadow on the left, the doctor ordered a full-body scan. The results of that scan were more than suspicious. The monk's body was peppered with small masses for which there was no logical explanation except cancer. They were in his lungs, his bones, and his liver.

This was a 60-year-old vegetarian who'd never smoked, who never drank alcohol, who spent his days in quiet contemplation and prayer.

I explained the monk's condition—cancer of the lung, metastasized throughout the body—and the futility of surgical intervention because it was so widespread. The translator conveyed my words carefully.

The monk watched each of us in turn as we spoke, his face relaxed, his expression neutral. I worried something might be lost in translation—that he might be missing some details, though the big picture was really the most important thing.

When I finished speaking, he spoke just a few words to the translator and then nodded to me and said, in soft, careful English, "I accept what is."

The range of reactions I see in patients grappling with new diagnoses runs the full gamut of human emotion, but this was the most unfazed response I'd ever heard. There was no indication the monk was stifling other emotions, that he was grieving, that he was shocked or angry or bitter or afraid. Just acceptance. As if I'd told him it was going to rain.

After this acknowledgment I laid out his limited treatment options and the reasonable chances of their success. The specific variety of his lung cancer was unresponsive to any as-yet-invented biologic or immunologic treatment. It was often resistant to even harsh chemotherapy regimens. We could try, though, to arrest the distant spread, to push it back. I would review all the relevant clinical trials to find anything for which he might be a candidate. He could opt for palliative chemo as well, relying on treatments to stave off the disease temporarily so he'd have more time and fewer symptoms.

I asked if he had questions, and he shook his head. *No, thank you, doctor.* And then he smiled at me—a kind, encouraging smile that made me feel the way I did when I was a kid and my dad would ruffle my hair or my grandmother would pat my hand and tell me she was proud.

I felt grateful and confused. How could a stranger make me feel that way? And why wasn't this man even a little bit upset by the news he was receiving? I was a bundle of nerves giving it, and he was serene.

Turning to the translator, I said I admired the monk's peaceful demeanor, and that I wondered how he was holding up so well.

The monk replied back through our intermediary, saying, "I love all of nature."

I thought I caught an emphasis on *all*, but maybe it was the translator's?

I took a step toward the door, but there was a question I couldn't leave unasked.

"The cancer?" I asked, thinking I must have misunderstood. *All* of nature?

He nodded and gave me another beatific smile.

"Yes," he said. "All is love."

With gentle urging, the monk chose to accept a short course of chemotherapy, and so a few days later he was comfortably tucked into a recliner in the treatment room, hooked up to an IV, peacefully napping. The sun through the window lit his face, giving him more than a little of the appearance of an angel. Other patients and their family members read and watched television nearby, occasionally stealing furtive glances at this man who looked as if he'd drifted in from another world.

I found time to visit the treatment room each time he was there, looking forward to being in his presence, if only for a few minutes. A high-strung, stressed-out guy like me had a lot to learn from a man like this, one who seemed able to transcend the drama of the moment, of this whole stage of his life.

I wasn't the only one. Other doctors, nurses, and members of our staff seemed to feel the same draw. No one wanted to disturb the monk, but everyone wanted to be near him. His presence was soothing, or grounding, or something. I'd been studying religion and meditation and all kinds of mind–body healing since my undergrad years, but I was at a loss to put my finger on exactly what was happening. My best guess is that this man had an aura that was a balm to my colleagues and me, setting us at ease just by being near it.

Four infusions and 12 weeks later, when the monk's next scan showed little change, I suggested an adjustment to the regimen, adding another chemical element to amplify the first.

He declined. "It is not necessary," the translator said for him. "I accept what is, but I thank you, doctor."

On his way out of the office, he stopped and rested his hand on mine, then gave a little bow and walked out the door.

He made it look so easy. The monk's total acceptance of a disease progression that could only end in his death pulled me up short.

♡

Not once in the time I was treating him did the monk or his translator ask about the origin of his disease. They didn't question why he would be afflicted by this particular cancer, which impacts people who smoke widely disproportionate to the general population.

I think he intuitively knew it didn't matter.

It made me ashamed of my ridiculous reaction to my skin cancer, trying to blame it on my life or my character or my attitude. I had a long way to go to putting this rough patch in my life behind me, but that particular mistake was one I would never make again.

My brief time with the monk inspired me to face this troubling problem head-on with the men and women who come into my care burdened by negative self-directed emotions about their illness. Some feel they brought it on themselves, like I did. Some feel they somehow deserve to be sick. Some are ashamed because their diagnosis is a cancer that the unknowing public tends to think is the result of poor or risky health or lifestyle choices. The monk—perhaps the most clean-living person I have treated in my entire career—never questioned. And starting with his case, I decided to make it a point to reassure each patient that he or she did not cause the cancer, did not invite it, and does not deserve it. There is zero room for the blame game in oncology—it's an unproductive and painful path to pursue and no good ever comes of it once someone has been diagnosed.

The monk's illness was an affirmation of the fact that disease can turn up any place, any time, in any host. Can you live your life in ways that are preventive? Absolutely, and please do it! Is there any sure thing? No, there's not. Does it matter what you did or didn't do in the past once you reach my office? No. From the moment of your diagnosis, you owe it to yourself and to the people who love you to live in the present and look to the future. The day you meet your oncologist for the first time may be the most appropriate day of your life to choose to dismiss the past, set it adrift, and not expend any of your precious energy looking back.

I accept what is was a worthy mantra, one I adopted and one that I share often.

CHAPTER 9

TRUE COLORS

*I was about to give up when I heard a footstep
And saw an inkling of a path.
Another had walked the trail up this mountain.
Eyes on my feet, I willed them forward.
Make a path; make a difference.*

— *DAILY DOSE*, AUGUST 30, 2019

Facing a new cancer diagnosis can feel like standing at the bottom of a steep, rocky mountain, staring up, thinking that the journey is impossible.

In an effort to try to regain control of my work and my health, I aligned with a group of my co-workers to found a new cancer treatment center. None of us had all the answers, but we were determined to find a healthier, kinder balance for our patients and ourselves. We wanted to be part of a group where everyone embraced the concept of being a team to help our patients—rather than one where we were essentially pitted against one another to gain and keep them. We wanted to foster an environment that was welcoming and nurturing, one where we could embrace complementary therapies. We wanted our patients to feel at home, and so we prepared our new office space with that in mind in every choice from the furniture to the artwork to the treatment room that was meant to have the feel of a coffeehouse.

There's only so much you can do to dress up an oncology office, but each choice was made with warm and honest intentions for our patients, and that mattered to me.

An even more important aspect of the change for me was the sense of ownership I felt in the new practice. I would not be along for the ride in another physician's practice. The patients would be *my* patients. I would be on the line, and I'd be able to create the kinds of relationships I'd dreamed of when I left Georgetown—relationships where I could build trust and bonds, where I could put in as much time as I saw fit. It was the first time in my career that the buck stopped with me, and I was eager and ready to take on that responsibility.

I believed in myself, in my partners, in the practice and the central tenets we'd agreed on from the beginning. Unfortunately, deep down, my guts were less confident. The pressure I felt to succeed and the stress that grew from that manifested itself in yet more medical issues. I was diagnosed with prostatitis and ulcerative colitis. My own roster of doctors included a rheumatologist, a neurologist, a pulmonologist, a dermatologist, a urologist, and a GI specialist. I couldn't sleep, and I couldn't get away from the pain in my muscles, my head, and my guts.

The occasion of what I honestly believed would be the start of a bright new professional future was shadowed by my body becoming a bundle of stress-induced ailments.

And then in December of 2006, in an attempt to circumvent a migraine, I took an over-the-counter pain reliever. Within an hour my heart was racing and my left arm and hand were numb. I lost vision in my left eye, as if a shade had closed over it. I thought I was having a stroke, and I raced straight to the emergency room. I was 36 years old, and that night I thought I was going to die.

After an MRI and a battery of blood tests, the diagnosis was an atypical migraine manifesting through left-side numbness and temporary blindness. The translation I heard was this: *Go home, Steven. Get some sleep. Eat better. Breathe. Get your shit together.* I knew extricating myself from that first, oppressive office had been key to getting my life on track, but clearly I still had work to do.

♡

It was in these early days of the new practice that I met a patient who would poignantly remind me why I'd chosen oncology, how blessed I was in my professional life, and of how little consequence my personal worries really were.

Clara was 20 years old when she went to the emergency room with excruciating back pain. Her family had put the visit off as long as they could, hoping she had just pulled or strained a muscle and would heal on her own. The pain kept getting worse, though, and they finally caved and asked for help.

In the ER the attending physician knew something was seriously wrong. Patients as young as Clara without chronic conditions rarely arrive in such extreme discomfort with no obvious injury or infection. She winced and writhed and her blood pressure spiked as she curled into the fetal position on a hospital bed and rode out waves of pain. A CT scan was ordered, and when the preliminary radiology report came back, the doctor requested an oncology consult and got me.

At my computer I read the report and opened the image file. All along Clara's spine, long, horrendous lesions shadowed her bones, insinuating themselves into her frame. In the middle of her chest, one of the masses had significantly eroded tissue and bone, and I wondered how she'd managed to walk into the ER under her own steam.

I ordered pain medication and reviewed her history. I wanted to be wrong, but after considering her record, I suspected that despite her age, Clara was suffering from a rare pediatric cancer.

Less than 24 hours later, it was confirmed. She had a form of Ewing's sarcoma, an aggressive bone tumor. It was a disease I knew by its terrible reputation, but not one I had treated because most of its victims are children younger than 15.

Because it commonly has micrometastases—tiny pockets of cancerous cells that spread through the body through the circulatory and lymphatic systems—the usual protocol for Ewing's is chemotherapy first, then surgery. The goal is for the chemo to seek and destroy as much of the cancer as possible and shrink the tumor (in this case multiple tumors) before surgery.

But Clara had to go straight to the OR. She was in too much pain, the tumors so far gone that permanent damage to her spinal cord would be inevitable without intervention. Her spine needed to be stabilized. She'd already lost some use of one arm, and waiting for chemo to do its work could cost her significantly more precious motor function.

Of course there was a catch: Clara was an undocumented immigrant with no insurance. Anything that was going to be done for her at the hospital would have to be done through her emergency room admission. She was ineligible for nonemergency care. Clara had been brought to the U.S. illegally with a family member as a young child, and now she was on the verge of being discharged with a host of deadly tumors growing on her bones because she didn't have a Social Security number.

The medical team at the hospital didn't want that to happen, and neither did I.

This was a patient who needed life-saving care, and she deserved to be in the care of someone who specialized in her condition. I got on the phone and called the nearest expert in Ewing's and asked if he would take her case. The answer was an apologetic but firm no. I called a specialist in Los Angeles, one in Sacramento, one in Seattle—working my way farther from San Diego, but getting the same response from each physician and office.

I'm sorry, but we can't take her without insurance.

By the time my calls reached the East Coast, I realized I was wasting precious time. This wasn't going to happen, and the patient was running out the clock on her ER stay. And so despite the twin facts that I was not the seasoned Ewing's expert she deserved and that our fledgling practice was not yet on solid footing (or anywhere near it), Clara became, by default, my patient.

To their credit the hospital staff was able to arrange, straight from the ER, the neurosurgery she needed to remove the tumor impinging her spinal cord. Once she was stable, they sent her home with her discharge instructions and my name, office address, and phone number.

♡

Here's what I believed then and know at this writing: the absolute worst things in the world of medical treatment happen when critical health decisions are made based on money. It's terrible in public and nonprofit care and even worse in private practice. I've had patients say, *Well, if that's what it's going to cost, I can't do it* or *I'm not going to bankrupt my family for this treatment.* Or they'll choose a lesser treatment.

Everything about cancer treatment—the pills, the infusions, the scans, the surgeries—it's all expensive, and the financial toxicity can take a huge toll on people's lives.

This was my first true taste of just how ugly and embittering the system can be, and at the center of the story was a young woman who was barely past childhood, randomly afflicted with a rare and deadly disease that just might be treatable.

She had her whole life ahead of her; or she might not.

At this writing there is no way around this truth, though heaven knows there are countless doctors and nurses, administrators and caregivers who try to find one. In our practice today, we have a team member whose primary focus is dedicated to reducing financial toxicity, working tirelessly to try to find grants and co-pay assistance, going toe-to-toe with insurance companies denying treatment, wrangling cost reductions on equipment and medications and treatments for our patients. Sometimes it's a losing battle, and sometimes she comes in like our very own white knight with a solution that helps.

The entire model is precarious, and if it collapses before we can fix it, it will pull countless patients down with it.

The first to fall will be patients like Clara, who have absolutely no cards to play within the system.

♡

The first time Clara came to the office after her surgery was also the first time I got a sense of her presence in the world, and it was tiny. She was frail and scared, her huge green eyes ringed with dark circles. She'd been through a traumatic ordeal, and her fear permeated the room. She came from a big, close-knit family, and her parents and siblings and grandmother all squeezed into the room, trying to understand what would happen next.

She had come in carrying a music player, so I asked, in my so-so Spanish, about her favorite music.

"*¿Cantas una canción favorita?*" *Do you sing a favorite song?*

Obviously surprised to be talking about anything but cancer, Clara smiled shyly and nodded.

"Cyndi Lauper," she said.

"Oh, you're an 80s girl!? *¿Cuál canción?" Which song?*

When she didn't answer right away, I sang the title lines of the tracks that came to mind, gauging her interest. The grandmother gave me a withering look, but she said nothing, waiting to see where this was going.

"I see your true colors shining through?"

"If you're lost you can look and you will find me?"

And then, figuring I had nothing to lose, I went for the laugh, bobbing my head and crowing, *"Ooooh girls just wanna have fu-un!"*

Clara giggled, then surprised me by singing back to me, in a perfectly Lauper-esque imitation, *"Lying in my bed I hear the clock tick and think of you . . ."*

"Oh, *that* one! That's a beauty—'Time After Time.'"

We sang a couple lines, and I suggested that, if it was okay with Clara, maybe that could be our song. We were going to be seeing a lot of each other and it would be great for us to have one.

After that we turned to the matter at hand—her treatment. The form Clara's disease had taken is one of its most vile—one that erodes away the spines of children. To have any chance of beating it, she'd need radiation and then many months of chemotherapy. We talked about the medications and their side effects, the support the office could provide, and how important it would be for each treatment to be given on time. Sticking to the regimen would be a huge commitment, because before she felt better she was likely to feel worse. For just a moment, I tuned out every other presence in the room and focused squarely on my patient.

"We are at the bottom of a tall mountain," I said in careful Spanish, "but we're going to climb together."

The first obstacle on my end of the equation was getting the drugs. There was no chance Clara or her family could afford them without insurance—almost no one can. With nowhere else to turn, I called the pharmaceutical company and asked what they could do. Their representative said she'd call me back. I waited two days before finally getting a call, but it was worth it: the company had agreed to donate the medicine. That was an ironic victory—being gifted a harsh regimen that would weaken and sicken Clara almost immediately after her first treatment and leave her diminished for the long haul. Next I called a radiology company that did scans for many of my patients, working my way up the phone chain until finally I got the CEO. I pointed out that my patients generated a lot of business for his company—most of it paid by their insurance. This patient didn't have a safety net. She would need scans every three months, probably for a long time, and I'd like the company to donate those scans.

To my surprise and gratitude, he agreed.

Clara's family rallied around her throughout her treatment. Different family members came to sit with her during chemo—sometimes her mother, sometimes a sister or brother or aunt. She became a favorite with the nurses. I think we all saw in her someone in our own lives—daughters, little sisters, nieces. All those girls in their teens and twenties, just getting their first taste of freedom, stepping out, trusting, into the big world. We wanted that for Clara too.

When she lost all her hair, she decided to own it rather than wear a wig, and she sported a ball cap someone had given her that said *Fuck Cancer* to her chemo sessions. She never complained, even when she became so thin and sick it seemed like even her hat was too big to fit anymore. The lack of protest wasn't necessarily a good thing, because it made me worry she might lose her will to fight. One morning as

I listened to her lungs, she leaned forward, almost resting her head on my chest, and I reflexively pulled her closer and gently hugged her. I thought of my own baby girls—of their healthy hearts and growing bodies and inquisitive minds. They were everything to me, and I knew this sweet, vulnerable barely-out-of-childhood woman held all that excitement and promise for her own family.

As I walked out of her room, I sang a line back to her from our song. *"If you're lost you can look and you will find me, time after time . . ."* In the hall I said a silent, fervent prayer that this girl would make it through her treatment; that she'd get a chance to live.

♡

Some days Clara sat silent, curled in her recliner, napping on and off while her chemo infusion dripped slowly into the medical port in her chest. Other days she played cards with her *tia* or sister or mom. One morning her nurse brought in a coloring book—one of the ones designed for adults and full of intricate op-arty sketches—and a box of colored pencils, and Clara spent hours hunched over the pages, filling in the tiny boxes. Her petite frame and her vulnerability sometimes made her appear childlike, but her apprehensions were those of an adult. She worried about her family and the emotional and financial toll her care was taking on them. She worried about whether she'd be able to have children. She worried about whether she'd ever be able to live a normal life again—to do all the things 20-year-olds do.

Her family was remarkably supportive. I'm not sure I ever once saw Clara alone, and when she had a full-body scan three months into her treatment, several of them crowded into the exam room to hear the results. The grandmother bowed her head, softly, fervently praying. An uncle bent and re-bent the brim of a baseball hat with both hands, his nervous energy obvious and contagious. Clara's sister held her hand.

Clara, gaunt and bald, her green eyes sunken and flat, looked at me. She'd been through so much since that initial trip to the ER, and each step of her treatment thus far had taken a visible toll on her fragile body. My mind jumped back to the first day of my fellowship, to *chemotherapy is a loaded gun*, and I felt awed by how strong Clara had been so far—and deeply apprehensive about how far she had to go.

"*Tio E.?*" she asked, using the honorary nickname she'd given me a few weeks in. *Uncle E.?*

The first time she'd said it, I'd melted.

"It's working," I said, focusing on her first and then nodding to each family member in turn. "The tumors are shrinking, changing slowly. The chemo is pushing them out, but it is going to take time, months more, before we can know if they will go away completely."

I caught the grandmother's eye and repeated the news, significantly simplified, in Spanish. "*Es bueno,*" I concluded, "*pero necesitamos mas.*" *We need more.* Tears slipped from the corners of her eyes.

"*Gracias a Dios,*" she said. *Thank God.*

♡

Clara was a fixture in our office, showing up every two weeks, month after month. Anyone who has ever experienced one of these regimens or taken care of someone going through it knows what a roller coaster of awfulness it is— each treatment knocks you on your ass, and just about the time you begin to feel better, the next one is due. It is discouraging at best. Some patients find ways to schedule a little time at the end of each cycle for R&R or family time or just to do something fun. But for a patient like Clara, with such a long course of treatment, the impacts were also cumulative, wearing her down not just in a regular biweekly cycle, but over the long haul as well.

My own health issues continued to fester and seemingly compound themselves, and I stocked a drawer in my desk with an overflowing stash of creams, inhalers, antacids, and over-the-counter pain meds. But I was reminded every day, and especially every other week when Clara showed up for treatment, that my life was blessed, that my problems were small-scale, and that my patients were counting on me to keep it together.

Over months, even with cost of the scans and her meds covered, Clara's bills added up. The office received small checks and envelopes containing cash with her name on them, and our staff began to realize there was a wide net of family and friends chipping in to help. One day I asked Clara about it, saying, "A lot of people must love you," and she told me more than 50 friends and family members had contributed to her care.

"I can never repay that," she said.

"Nobody wants to see you pay a debt, Clara," I said. "They want to see you walk out of here healthy. Maybe even see you have some fun."

As the months went on, Clara's tumors continued to shrink, but her treatments took a toll. At home she was sick to her stomach and listless. On the days she couldn't even keep water down, her mother brought her to the office for IV fluids. Her blood pressure dropped, and we knew her heart was being strained by her meds. Family members and I made lists of things Clara might be able to eat, concocting recipes for milkshakes with extra protein, extra calcium, extra of any nutrient we could figure out how to include.

And then, finally, after a year of grueling, grinding treatments, Clara's scan came back NED: no evidence of disease. I called her from the office the minute the news came through, and could hear her alternately crying and shouting on the other end of the line.

The practice team threw a party at the office to celebrate the remission, with cake and tears of joy all around. I made a goofy attempt to salsa dance into the room and Clara gamely tried to match my steps. We sang along with Kool and the Gang's "Celebration" and our song, "Time After Time." Clara pretended to have a microphone, and I leaned in to share it with her on the chorus.

Clara had endured the longest chemotherapy regimen our practice had ever given a patient—bullet after bullet after bullet—and she had survived. It was the most gratifying day of my career so far, one I would use as a touchpoint for years to come at times when things looked bleak.

Clara's remission hadn't come without a price. She had sacrificed most of a year of her life. She would have lasting neuropathy and a long road back to a healthy weight. She would likely never be able to conceive a child. She would always have to live with the possibility of recurrence. But that day, she hugged the nurses who had treated her like family and she threw her arms around me, calling me *Tio*. She went home cancer free to start living her second chance.

♡

Clara was the first patient with whom I likened fighting cancer to hiking, but since then I often tell my patients that they are about to climb a mountain—Everest, even—and that they don't have to go alone.

"I'll be your Sherpa, because I've been there before," I say, only half joking. "We'll hike it together."

Coping with cancer and fighting back against it is a mountain for every patient and for every family. No good comes of just standing at the bottom staring up. What does work is setting small goals and taking steady steps—laying out the route, taking in the lay of the land, climbing over the first rise, stopping to rest, setting out again to cover a little more ground. No matter the ultimate destination of your journey, it is a massive undertaking. And even when you have people to love you to lean on, it's a lonely one. You need to be able to trust your medical team to be experienced, steadfast, and protective guides—step after step after step.

Clara made it all the way to the top of that mountain, and she was able to stand there and look out at the view, at the future on her horizon. On that last day of her treatment, I hoped and prayed she'd be up there for a long, long time, living the healthy, happy life for which she'd fought so valiantly.

CHAPTER 10

IT HAD
TO BE YOU

If you can't take care of yourself,
How will you take care of us?

— *Daily Dose*, November 7, 2019

One of my most beloved patients at this time was a woman who was Clara's polar opposite—a confident, boisterous elderly lady named Flavie who had stage IV lung cancer. For Flavie, it was all *c'est la vie*—nothing ruffled her. I loved to listen to her stories of being a dancer in Vegas and of giving her daughters childhoods full of love and light. Her husband had died young, so she had done it alone, and she was proud of that. She referred to her girls—mothers themselves by then—as her tour de force.

Flavie was charismatic and stylish—she had the undeniable presence of a performer. She had bright blue-green eyes, perfect posture, and the raspy voice of a longtime smoker. I never saw her when she wasn't wearing an eye-catching, ultra-feminine outfit or accessory, even when she was in the hospital. On a good day, she'd turn up in my office in a smart, Chanel-esque suit, or a turtleneck and capri pants like an octogenarian Audrey Hepburn. Many of my patients—and I, for that matter—found ourselves too busy, too tired, too sick, or just too focused on other things to put in the kind of effort that obviously went into her appearance, but it was second nature to Flavie. Even when she didn't feel well enough to put together a full ensemble, she'd wear a wide-brimmed hat, or a pair of Jackie O.–style sunglasses, or a silk scarf knotted loosely at her neck—always something that made her stand out.

In the hospital, where she spent some time due to the chemotherapy complications of fever, low blood counts, and bronchitis, she'd wear the scarf over her head, expertly tied at the nape of her neck, or feathered slippers, or a satin robe over her standard-issue gown. No matter where you found her, Flavie had style.

One morning when I visited her on rounds, I poked my head in quietly, not wanting to wake her if she was sleeping. The IV antibiotics were helping, but she was still weak and needed to rest. As it turned out, she wasn't too groggy to perk up when she saw me.

"Good morning, Dr. E.!" she exclaimed in her cheerful, raspy voice, setting down her book, sitting tall, and giving me a wink. Even in a hospital bed, she had ramrod posture.

I asked how she was feeling and got the usual—*okay, a little old*. And then the zinger, "But how are *you*?" she said. "Because you look like shit today."

Did I mention she had a fondness for colorful language? This too was part of her charm, because it was (almost) always done in a spirit of fun. She clearly knew peppering her speech would keep her audience attentive—even when it was just her doctor, in the hospital, at 7:00 on a Tuesday morning.

I'd barely slept, skipped the gym, choked down a coffee, and was slogging through my rounds and appointments with my guts in knots. I didn't need anyone to tell me I looked awful—I felt it. Still, I paused to remember if I'd taken my morning meds, then focused on the new blood work numbers in Flavie's chart.

"I'm fine," I said, not looking up, "just busy."

"*Really,* Dr. E.?" She scrutinized my face, then shook her head. "Bullshit. If you can't take care of yourself, how will you take care of us?"

"I'm not sure what you mean," I lied, reminding myself that I loved this prying old lady. She frequently called me *kid* and kept a steady stream of encouragement coming my way during her appointments. It sometimes felt like she was training me for a marathon rather than allowing me to treat her for a terminal disease. Even as I was trying to get caught up on how *she* was feeling, she'd ask about my vitamin regimen or my sleep schedule, or remark that I looked pale. On her way out, she'd look back over her shoulder and offer a final note of encouragement. "Great job today," she called one afternoon. And on another, "Now don't forget to get a good lunch!"

Flavie had made it clear from her first visit that she was only accepting treatment at her daughters' insistence—that she wasn't really interested in all the fuss that came with it. She'd downplay even severe symptoms if I didn't push her to let me help with them. ("How's the nausea?" I asked one day. "I was never a big eater anyway," she replied.)

But on this day, she wasn't in an encouraging mood so much as she was in one to take me to task. "*I don't know what you mean,*" she mimicked, wagging a finger at me. "You know *exactly* what I mean. I mean Take. Care. Of. Yourself."

I sighed and turned back to the chart. "Okay, Flav, but let's talk about you. How are *you* feeling today? Because you look fabulous, but your white counts are still low."

She looked at me like I was daft. "White counts?" she scoffed. "Is that all you want to talk about? Dr. E., you've got to have some fun in your life."

And then she said, "How about a dance? That'll make us both feel better."

I hesitated, then opened my mouth to decline, but she was already struggling to her feet, humming "It Had to Be You." Hustling to her side, I reached out to make sure she wouldn't fall. She slid her feet into her bright pink slippers, and I steadied her before putting one hand at her waist and one on her shoulder.

Her voice was shaky but pitch-perfect as she sang, "*I wandered around and finally found somebody who . . .*" She paused to stage-whisper at me, "SING!"

As we twirled slowly around the hospital room singing our duet, I felt my stress start to slip. Flavie was 84 years old, dying of lung cancer, and trailing an IV and a heart monitor; but she was defiantly joyful, her voice lifting as she looked me in the eye and sang, "*With all your faults, I love you still.*" I was 37, in my white coat and stethoscope, a knotted-up stress ball with colitis and vertigo and chronic fatigue—a mess.

In that moment instead of mentally cataloging how I was feeling, where I had to be next, and how many appointments I had ahead, I found myself laughing and singing along, caught up in the unexpectedly joyful moment. There was something about being with Flavie that made me feel like maybe I *was* training for a marathon of sorts—that perhaps I was just warming up, still short of my potential. As I gently danced her back toward her bed and helped her settle under the quilt she'd brought from home, I found myself thinking, *Maybe I'm doing this all wrong.* I wondered if maybe that dance, that connection, might be meaningful beyond the room and the hospital and this lovely, feisty patient who seemed to be daring me to be better. The burnout I'd been experiencing for years eased just long enough for me to think, with unexpected clarity, *If I start taking ownership of my practice of medicine right now, I might be able to make this right . . . I can still be the doctor I want to be.*

I knew my heart was in the right place, but I had been struggling to keep my life from cracking under the pressure of my work for far too long.

I wondered if I could do for my patients what Flavie was doing for me. What if I could find a way to give them moments like this, reminding them of who they were deep down, beyond the reach of the cancer?

There must have been something powerful in that pure, joyful moment with Flavie that sparked a change in me, because I left her room willing to try.

♡

When I think of Flavie now, it is with gratitude and love. There was magic in our dance that day. Her kindness, her candor, her unsteady steps, and her ringing, melodic voice are all still with me, still lift me. So often I meet cancer patients who feel diminished. They're sick, they're shrinking as they lose weight, they struggle with bearing the scars of their surgeries and treatments. But Flavie, without any coaching, was larger than life, even in her illness. She somehow managed to be, in her eighth decade, as open and opinionated, kind and graceful and musical as she'd ever been in her life. If I could help my patients move away from the shadows of disease and treatment—back toward the core of who they were before and would be after—I could make a difference.

I started thinking of it as the "Flavie effect." How could I bring the kind of immediate, unfettered connection and joy she brought me to my patients? I was determined to figure it out.

CHAPTER 11

BORN TO RUN

One little word
Can mean the world,
Can rock someone's world,
Can change someone's world.

— *Daily Dose*, December 11, 2019

During the time that Flavie was under my care, I'd entered an essay contest hosted by Peter Himmelman, whose songwriting inspired me and whose music soothed me after many a dark, draining day in med school. He'd invited fans to describe how his music had touched their lives, and I sent a letter about the way his songs helped me through med school, calling it "Mission of My Medicine," after Peter's song "Mission of My Soul."

I won! The prize was a personal song from Peter, one he would write just for me. I took winning as a sign that I should listen to Flavie's assessment, trust my gut, and get to work figuring out how to bring more positivity and joy to my practice. Another quick and intense connection with a patient over a shared love of a musician brought me back to music as the key.

♡

On the same day as my dance with Flavie, Jason came to me with colon cancer that had spread to his liver—a full-blown stage IV. He was so thin and weak he struggled to make it from the waiting room to the exam table that first day. Once there he told me about his career as a college professor and his passion for researching and writing about history. We talked about his goals for treatment. (*A cure would be ideal,* he said diplomatically, *but being well enough to get back to work for a while would be good too.*) Then he told me he was in possession of tickets to a sold-out Springsteen show in a few months' time, and that he really did not want to miss his chance to hear The Boss.

Ah, Springsteen. I rolled closer on my stool and we spent the next 10 minutes debating which album was his best, who were our favorite band members, and what we wouldn't give to be at one of those New Jersey bars where the E Street Band showed up unannounced and played one of their famously epic concerts.

As we spoke, the man who had come into the room hobbled and heartsick became more animated, caught up in our shared excitement about the music we both loved. For just a few moments, I glimpsed how he must have carried himself before he'd begun to lose weight—first 10 pounds, then 10 more and yet 10 more—before he'd noticed dark blood in his stools, before he'd begun to feel overwhelmingly tired, and before his skin had taken on the telltale tinge of yellow that told his family doctor something was seriously wrong. The vibrant, clever, strong man was still within him, just hidden by the disease.

A stage IV diagnosis of any kind is terrifying, and in the not-so-distant past it was typically a death sentence. Jason was operating on the assumption that he was dying and he was making his final plans. I could not possibly promise him a positive outcome, but I was able to offer a glimmer of hope.

Despite his ominous diagnosis, the oncologists' toolbox for pushing back against this particular colon cancer, even with its far-reaching spread, was well-stocked. Jason wasn't a candidate for surgical resection, but he had options. He fit the criteria to have the traditional chemotherapy regimen for his disease augmented by Avastin—a rising star drug that effectively starves tumors of blood supply.

Jason seemed confused and even a little offended by my words. Like most patients, he'd been reading about his condition. As a skilled researcher, he'd done a deep dive. What he'd encountered had been decades of studies suggesting he probably had less than a year to live. As I was trying to read his irritation, he spelled it out.

"Please don't toy with me," he said. "I want the truth. I want to be able to prepare, and I need to be honest with my family."

Sometimes I forget that this happens—that people in the medical world (or on the fringes of it) peddle false hope. It's not something I do, nor do my partners. The truth can be brutal, but it is necessary, and every patient deserves to be respected enough to hear it straight and unvarnished from his or her oncologist. The thing was, especially in this particular case, the hope was real.

"I am never, ever gonna sugarcoat your condition," I told him, catching his gaze and holding it. "Without treatment, everything you've been reading is true. With only the treatment that was available ten years ago? Still true. But things are changing every day, and the cancer in your body is one I have seen go into complete remission.

"That's not any kind of promise," I continued. "It's way too soon to know how this ends, whether you and I will be back here in six or eight months talking about how to make you comfortable, or in two years talking about what concerts we've seen and who's the greatest guitarist of all time."

I flipped open a tablet and spun my stool so we could look at it together. "I know you're going to keep reading about this," I said. "I'd do the same. But I want you to stop looking at any studies that were published more than a year ago. Okay?"

He nodded.

"Even then, you're not going to be reading the latest, because treatment development and studies and outcomes and writing and reviewing and submitting for publication—it all takes time. As you read I hope you'll keep in mind that I believe the day is coming when we'll be talking about cases like yours not in terms of one-year survival, but three, and then five, and then ten. Someday maybe it'll be longer."

After we talked, we looked at some study data together and laid out the plan for the treatment that would tie us together for the coming months. In addition to the medical interventions, I also recommended a protein shake I'd been tinkering with—a recipe to help patients who were struggling to maintain weight.

That night at home, I took the Ovation Legend from its stand in the corner for the first time in months and picked out the chords of "Born to Run." I cuddled my baby girls and sat down to dinner with my beautiful, exhausted wife and held her hand. I felt better than I had in a long time. Hungry and tired, but not sick or stressed out.

Lying in bed I let the Springsteen lyrics play in my head, my fingers working the chords even without the guitar.

I fell asleep thinking how great it had felt to play again, even for a few minutes. How grateful I was to live in the same time as The Boss. How much I wanted to be able to capture the optimism of the past few days of my life and share them with the cancer patients in my care.

In the morning I scooped up the guitar on my way to the car and settled it in the passenger seat. In the office parking lot, I looked over at it, thought, *Why not?,* and carried it inside. After seeing my morning patients, I carried it to the treatment room, feeling as conspicuous in the hall as if I'd been riding a horse or waving a giant flag.

Relax, Steven, I muttered. *You've done this before.*

At the door I surveyed the patients hooked up to IV drips, the family members who sat with them, and the nurses who worked the room, checking ports and making notes, meting out anti-nausea meds and offering water and cookies and blankets and reassurance. I asked if anyone would mind if I played a few songs and got no objections. So I pulled up a straight-backed chair, positioning myself so I wouldn't disrupt the flow of traffic in and out of the room or to and from the bathroom.

What followed was perhaps the most awkward concert of all time—me playing a few Adam Sandler-esque ditties to polite laughter and a couple wan smiles. I asked one elderly patient named Bette, who seemed to be amused, what her favorite thing was. She played along, answering, "I've got six dogs and three cats!" So I cleared my throat and said, with mock pretension, "This song is called 'Six Dogs and Three Cats,' and I wrote it for Bette." Strumming a tune consisting of just a couple chords, I rambled on about pets and Bettes. I felt ridiculously vulnerable, playing the musical clown, but when I looked around the room, the patients made my vulnerability seem trite. There they sat, sleeves rolled up for needles or shirts unbuttoned to expose Mediports, letting the poison my colleagues and I had carefully selected drip into their veins. Bette, who'd lost her hair and 25 pounds so far, sat bundled under a sweater and a blanket. I realized I was perhaps the least vulnerable person in the room, and since Bette was laughing, I kept playing.

That silly chemo concert was the first step in a sea change in my approach to medicine. Music, always at the periphery of my practice, took one giant step toward the center. Encouraged by the positivity breaking out my guitar brought to the room, I did it again a few days later, and a few days after that. The nurses said it brightened up the trenches. My partners didn't hesitate to throw their support behind the idea, high-fiving me in the hall and popping into the treatment room to say an encouraging word.

I started looking for other ways to connect on a more personal, less clinical level with my patients. I gave in to the simple human urge to hug distressed patients more often. I took a little more time with each to ask about their hobbies, their children, their favorite stories and songs. I sat beside them in the exam rooms and encouraged them to feel what they needed to feel—rage, sorrow, betrayal, frustration, confusion—until they'd expressed enough to make a little room for hope in whatever form I could give it to them. If they got better, I shared their joy. If they got sicker, I tried to get closer, rejecting the reflexive, self-preserving instinct to distance myself to spare some grief down the line. I had enough experience to know by then that if I was going to try to break down the wall between doctor and patient, I'd have to do it in sickness, in health, and also in death.

♡

Jason, in a realization of everything I'd hoped for him, became an Avastin champion. He went into remission, and he went back to work. There was no way to predict if it would last a year, or five or ten, but he reclaimed his life and was determined to live it fully. When I asked him about the Springsteen concert, he lit up, raving about the show.

He said, "I was alive!"

How often in your life do you hear anyone say *I am alive*? In oncology I hear it all the time. In conversations and in texts from patients: *I. Am. Alive. I was ALIVE today. I'm so alive!*

Some of these patients, like Jason, are celebrating a remission or a cure. Some know they are dying, and so *I am alive today* carries unspoken reservations about tomorrow. But all who speak these words are alive in ways too many of us forget to celebrate. They are *urgently* alive.

Feeling that way is a gift, an accomplishment, a transcendence. For my cancer patients, it almost inevitably means surviving or rising above pain—transforming that pain into something positive and electric and beautiful.

Springsteen sang about living with sadness, embracing madness, about being out on a wire and the ultimate walk in the sun. I have no reason to think he wrote "Born to Run" about cancer, but there it was, all the same: the desperation and pain and breakthrough that I was feeling and Jason was feeling, that so many of my patients were going through. It's impossible to tell another person how to get to that place of transcending pain, but by the end of the first months of schlepping my guitar to work, and remembering Flavie's admonishment to have a little fun, and literally wrapping my arms around my patients, I was there.

CHAPTER 12

GRACE

My heart sank.
I pictured my deathbed.
I considered who was there,
Appraised the feelings,
Reviewed my life,
Mulled my choices,
Deliberated my shoulda-woulda-couldas.
I saw my family,
Overwhelmed with connection.
My heart rose.
On my deathbed,
Nothing but love.

— DAILY DOSE, FEBRUARY 22, 2019

I wish I could say that every patient had the kind of response to treatment that Jason had, that the steps I was taking to improve my practice somehow changed the prognosis for everyone in my life. But that's not the way oncology works. Every day brings patients who are living and also patients who are dying.

We serve them equally. Because this is not intuitive or easy, I frequently renew my commitment to help patients die in comfort and with dignity, and strive to steer delicate family conversations back to patients' wishes again and again.

In many ways my patient Richard deserves the credit for teaching me to make peace with the times I am powerless to beat the cancer. He was a giant of a man with a strong handshake, a deep, gravelly voice, and a penchant for plaid shirts and blue jeans. Before he lost his beard to chemo, he'd looked like a modern-day Paul Bunyan.

His diagnosis was pancreatic cancer. It has a devastating prognosis and advances in its treatment have been painstakingly small and slow. At this writing it remains one of the most aggressive and treatment-resistant forms the phantom takes. I hope one day I can describe it differently and offer more and better options. Right now, though, it's critical to open parallel dialogues with families about chemotherapy, radiation, and surgery, and also about what the medical team can do to maximize each patient's quality of life. These conversations, often starting at the first appointment, must promise clear and honest communication and extend as much loving support as is humanly possible. A pancreatic cancer diagnosis creates an instant crisis; patients and their loved ones deserve every ounce of grace and kindness the medical world can provide.

Some pancreatic cancer patients arrive knowing only what they've been told in an emergency room, and they are traumatized by the shock of the diagnosis and the delivery of it in such fast-paced, often confusing environments. Even patients with glimmers of hope in their diagnoses—early detection, operable tumors, somewhat less aggressive neuro-endocrine tumors—often come into the oncology office for the first time feeling desperate and distraught. Googling statistics about the disease only makes things worse, especially when outdated data takes center stage. The whole thing can feel like one crushing blow after another.

Richard came at his disease from a different vantage point than most patients. He'd spent his entire career in a hospital, working as a radiation technologist, exacting information to help those who were suffering from the same disease that afflicted him. After he became my patient, we spoke at length about his diagnosis, his treatment options, and often about the strengths and limitations of the tools at our disposal to diagnose and treat cancer. Richard was well-read in the field and up on every new advance on the horizon. One day when our conversation touched on my feelings of futility in some cases, he reacted with surprise. He told me that in all his years in the radiology suite, he'd never thought to blame an oncologist for a patient's worsening tumors.

"Look, Dr. E.," he said as we reviewed his new scans together, me apologizing as we took them in from every angle, "I hate to break it to you, but you're not God. You don't get to choose who gets sick, or even who gets healed. None of us do. I know you're using all the tools you've got. If you measure your worth by who lives and who dies, this job is going to kill you."

I knew he was right, but I wondered aloud if there was really any better way to measure success for a doctor than survival—even for an oncologist.

"Of course there is," Richard said, shaking his head at me as if I'd overlooked the obvious. "There are plenty of better measures. Asking *Did he make it?* is way too simple. Look at any case; look at me. Now ask yourself: *Did I give this guy more time?* Yeah, you did—you are. *Did I help him understand his options?* You did that too. What about *Has this part of my patient's life—this HARD part of his life—been better with me than it would have been without me?*"

I waited for him to answer.

"You're damned right it has," he said. "C'mon, Doc. You have to know that."

I'm not especially insecure, but nearly every oncologist struggles with the questions Richard was asking. Many of us struggle with them every day. When I get a patient back with a recurrence, it's not just business as usual. It's time to dig and scrape and test and research and ask questions: *Is there anything new? Is anything working? Have I seen this before, and how did that turn out?* As a field we have a lot to work with these days. Through robotic and laparoscopic surgery, we have access to better and less invasive biopsies and excisions. We have tremendous advances in imaging. We have a whole new world of understanding, just in the last 20 years, of how we can examine the genes and proteins in a tumor and create targeted therapies that block its growth signals or destroy diseased cells outright. We have advanced genomic testing and tech companies dedicated to creating personalized combination therapies designed for each individual rather than for an entire population. Often the answer to *Is there anything new?* is *Yes*.

But sometimes it isn't. Sometimes we are at the end of the line in terms of treatment, and patients and families have hard decisions to make about what comes next.

That was the case for Richard, nearly a year after our conversation.

♡

We sat in his hospital room—Richard, his wife, their children, and I. He was 51, and his cancer had metastasized throughout his body. He was running out of time.

"We need a miracle," Eileen demanded. She was so distraught that I was struggling to help her comprehend Richard's diminishing options.

I put my hand on her shoulder, thinking of all the times I had been in a room with this family, of how I looked at Richard and saw a friend, a brother.

"Look, sometimes the miracle is not the chemo," I said. "It's the love you have for each other and for the children you have together. It's the life you built."

Richard had been dozing in the bed, but when he heard my words, his attention turned to me. He met my eyes, gave me a small nod.

"Tell me what's on your mind," I asked him. "Where are you with everything that's going on right now?'

"I just want to be comfortable," he answered.

Richard's children started to cry openly. Two of them were in college. The youngest was just 17. Their grief filled up the room. I could feel it in the air, mixed with the oxygen, stinging my eyes and lungs.

"I want him to have more chemo," Eileen said. "You must have something else."

My heart ached for her, for their entire family, but after so many lines of treatment, there were waning returns to any further chemo. If Richard truly wanted another bullet, I would comply, but I would not ask him to suffer more to appease anyone.

Richard understood exactly what was happening, I was certain. He'd conducted thousands of scans, seen the images on his computer screen, learned to read the odds.

"Tell me what you'd like right now," I asked him.

"I want to go quick," he said, speaking to me but fixing his eyes on his wife, "and have no pain." He reached for Eileen's hand and she moved to his side.

"Thank you for telling me," I replied. "We can do that. I can help you be comfortable."

After months of treatment and tests and respites that he used to spend time with his kids, his wife, and their close friends, Richard was done fighting. In that moment all I could do for him was help his family acknowledge the love in the room and open themselves to the possibility that after living a good life, and after making a valiant stand against the phantom, the thing he longed for now was a good death.

As I walked down the hall, leaving the family with their grief, I thought of my own wife and children, of how they rely on me to be mentally and physically healthy and strong. I vowed to try to judge myself in the future by Richard's generous measure of an oncologist's success. I don't have miracles at my disposal, but sometimes I can use the art and science of my practice to offer other, smaller blessings: hope, understanding, consolation, treatment, remission, and second chances in the form of precious time.

♡

It is the solemn responsibility of the oncologist to help each patient navigate the path he or she chooses through the disease. If you want to fight, we fight. If you want to choose a different path, we go that way. I make suggestions, lay out options, and never spare you the truth. And then, to the best of my ability, I embrace your marching orders.

One of the things that becomes clearest in engaging with patients and families and disease every day is that joy and beauty can share the same emotional space with excruciating pain. Martin Luther King, Jr., wrote, "Only when it is dark enough can you see the stars." Cancer is a pitch-dark, cold sky, but against its backdrop, the most spectacular constellations appear: families making peace; spouses rekindling love; simple and pure joys like sunshine and ice cream and fresh flowers and a child's hug. For the many patients who are cured and move on, those stars stay, radiant, sometimes for the rest of their lives. But for Richard, the stars—exquisite, priceless moments—instead became the foundation of a family's bittersweet memories, and an assurance that the love they shared would continue to shine in their lives even after he was gone.

CHAPTER 13

TEACHING ME

Don't wait.
Tell your people what you love about them
While they're alive,
While they can hear you.

— *DAILY DOSE*, APRIL 25, 2020

It took two very different men to make me realize that there was still a leap to be made as I brought music into my practice. Each of them left an indelible mark on my life that helped cement the importance of validating each individual, first as a person and only after that as a patient.

The first was Peter Himmelman, who sent the song he wrote for me as a prize soon after I won his contest. As an admirer of his songwriting for more than a decade, I was in awe of this honor. I'd been in the crowd at his shows, amazed at his ability to hold an audience spellbound. I'd spent time turning his richly woven lyrics over in my head, analyzing the words and phrases in just the right context to give them heft and complexity. I'd been a fan since my med school days, and being acknowledged by him in such a meaningful way felt like a nudge toward self-acceptance, productivity, and positivity. It also kept the guitar in my hands, inspiring me to practice and try out new melodies and riffs when I played in the treatment room. Those moments felt as though they were knitting the strands of music and healing in my life together into something stronger than either was alone.

A second powerful influence at this time was a patient named Chuck. He'd been a songwriter, performer, and instrumentalist for more than 40 years, and as we bonded over our shared love of melody and harmony, rhythm and blues, he inspired me to do something completely new.

Chuck was suffering from a rare and aggressive form of prostate cancer—one that almost always presents only after it is metastatic to lymph nodes, bones, or distant organs. Treatments for many cancers have evolved in leaps and bounds in recent decades, changing outcomes for countless patients, but for some, including this one, we still have a long way to go.

Treatment would give Chuck some quality time, but from the first time we met he seemed to intuitively know and accept that his life was on a different path. There's a Buddhist teaching that focuses on the idea that a glass is already broken—that everything in life is fragile and impermanent, so we must relish the time we have and accept that nothing lasts. For a man who had not yet reached retirement age, who adored his spouse, who was leading a rich, full life, Chuck was remarkably grounded in his own being in the face of such a devastating diagnosis. Even living with sorrow, he had the demeanor of a wise old soul.

During his treatment and palliative care, we often talked about music. Chuck's band had opened for the Rolling Stones in the 60s—a fact that gave him instant credibility with me (and almost everyone else he met). His Elvis- and Beatles-inspired band wore suits and skinny ties and even had a local radio hit.

In middle age he'd had a musical variety show in Vegas. He brought a hilarious (and dirty) ditty that had been part of his act to one of his appointments and I roared with laughter as he re-created it live.

Chuck said it had been the most wonderful ride, right up until a fan died in a drunk-driving accident following one of his shows. After that he'd lost his desire to play for big, boisterous crowds. At home he became depressed. His wife at first hinted, then pushed, then insisted he try teaching. And she was right; it revived him. By the time I met him, he'd taught a whole generation of kids from his community and moved on to teaching their children. He told me teaching had brought him back to life, and that he loved the idea of his legacy living on in all those piano students still playing after he was gone.

The idea of living on, of music living on, stuck with me. I thought about anthems and elegies, hymns and ribald lyrical tributes. It swept me back to childhood and the one passage from my parents' shelf of self-help books that I'd always carried with me: Wayne Dyer's admonition, *Don't die with your music still in you.*

♡

When Peter Himmelman sent the song he'd written for me, the lyrics said, *Doctor knows that music can soothe the soul . . . Doctor's got it all under control.* It was ironic that by the time I heard it, I was actually starting to feel like I was getting things under control for the first time in years. As I listened to it over and over again, I got caught up in the power of the song. There were so many melodies and lyrics that were meaningful to me, but this one was uniquely mine. It felt like something permanent and lasting about me and about my life.

Chuck was the first person I shared it with after my family. We listened to it together, and when the song ended, he said, "That is the most amazing gift. You'll have that forever."

That's the moment when a lot of what had been swimming around in my head since meeting him came together, when I knew what we should do.

"We could write one together, you and me. A song about you," I said, "about your story."

It was a little presumptuous of me to offer to co-write a song with a man who had such an impressive background in professional music, but he agreed right away. Outside of his appointments, we chatted on the phone about his career, his calling to teach, the moments he credited with helping him define his life.

Chuck was the more accomplished songwriter of the two of us, but he was coping with his illness and focusing on spending time with his family, so I took a stab at cobbling a song together from our brainstormed notes.

We called it "Teaching Me," and by the time I was ready to play it through the first time for Chuck at his home, he'd begun hospice care. This patient concert was different from the ones I'd been playing in the chemo room since my dance with Flavie. This time half my audience was on his deathbed, half was the spouse who would guard and treasure his legacy. I felt as though the weight of my worth in their lives was inextricably tied to the musical experiment we'd undertaken together. I'd played in countless rooms for far more people, but I was certain so much had never been riding on my performance before. Disappointing this person to whom I'd promised something special would be failure on a massive, consequential scale.

Still, there was no choice but to go forward. They were waiting. I strummed my guitar and sang about skinny ties and piano lessons and finding redemption in music, fighting to keep my voice even.

Chucky, it's time for the show
Where's your skinny tie?

Put your good suit on . . .

Chuck watched and listened, intent. When I caught his eye, he nodded, encouraging me to play on.

The whole performance ran about two minutes before I reached the final chorus and sang:

Time for a change,
Time to give back,
Guide a smaller hand.
Who will you be
When they see
You are teaching me?

Tears streamed down Chuck's face and his wife's. He reached out and grabbed my hand.

"You get me," he said. "It's such a validation."

And then he said, "Encore! C'mon! Play it again."

I got tears all over my Ovation Legend that day, and I knew I'd been a part of something positive and powerful.

♡

There's a phrase in oncology and in medicine in general that we're hearing a lot more in recent years: *illness identity.* It's how we talk about the way a patient self-identifies during times of illness compared to before and after. It doesn't always fall neatly within the dates of diagnosis and treatment—in fact, many patients continue to identify as the sick version of themselves long after they've reached remission or cure. It makes sense, especially when we're talking about cancer. It's a phantom that comes into your life and changes everything—your body, your relationships, your routine, how you feel about yourself, and what constitutes a good day or a bad day. Of course you don't stay the same. The form this phenomenon takes is different for each person—and at different stages for the same person as well. In all its forms, though, it can weigh heavily on the confidence and self-possession of patients and on their relationships.

One of the ways medical and psychological professionals sometimes assess illness identity is in terms of *engulfment*—how much a person's condition is wrapped up in the way they perceive themselves. It's a term that implies the possibility of drowning, and sometimes dealing with cancer can definitely feel like being caught in an overwhelming tide. On the other end of the spectrum is *enrichment*—a place and stage where a patient's illness leads to positive changes in relationships and self-perception. Those two experiences can be miles apart, but any gesture or insight that helps bridge the gap is a powerful tool.

One of the things Chuck and I discovered together was that songwriting was one of those tools. The process took him almost effortlessly back to his roots—to the core of his identity. We revisited his glory days, his crises, his most personal and meaningful accomplishments. While we were working on his song, he wasn't a patient, he was a fascinating, talented, generous man. The process put the "real" and fully realized person back at the front of his psyche, and mine. His word, *validation,* was precisely the right one. In fact, I later realized, that was our objective. At least for a little while, we had cast off the shadow and weight of Chuck's illness and focused instead on the unique, creative, consequential presence of the man. We weren't denying what he was going through, but we were honoring all of him that was greater and more.

It doesn't take writing a song to do this (although it is one great way). It takes stepping a little closer, asking questions, listening to answers, sharing photographs or stories or memories or plans for the future. It requires us to recognize that none of the range of our human emotions and experience falls away when we get sick. We're still funny, smart, kind—and also impatient, angry, and bored. Illness is a single facet of who we are, not its entirety. As friends, family, caregivers, and medical professionals, we owe it to the people we care about to be constantly mindful that a cancer diagnosis doesn't define them. Even when the world seems completely honed in on the disease, we can make a point to validate the whole, complicated, beautiful person.

♡

Months after I first played "Teaching Me" for Chuck, I played it again at his memorial service. It was a celebration of life held at the home of a family friend. Several of Chuck's students played favorites of the pieces he'd taught them, and then his widow asked me to play our song. As I strummed the guitar, a group of Chuck's students started singing along with the chorus, and then the whole room joined in. It was unlike any moment I'd ever experienced as a doctor or as a performer—the lyrics and melody Chuck and I conceived together took on a life of their own, evoking the man who was not there but who would somehow remain a part of everyone in the room.

Later, as I latched my guitar case, the host came over and shook my hand. "That was really something," he said. "Do you do this with all your patients?"

"This was my first," I told him. "But I think I'm going to start doing it a lot more."

CHAPTER 14

GENEROUS HEART

Life is a series of songs.
Some you like; others you don't.
You can't always get what you want.
It isn't as easy as Spotify.

What if we stop trying to get happiness on demand?
Be surprised,
Open to new possibilities,
New songs alongside our greatest hits.

Great music is like magic.
Hit shuffle.
Let it play.
Feel better.

— *Daily Dose*, April 2, 2019

Songwriting with Chuck was a revelation. My musical process had always been all about me—what I felt and needed to express and wanted to be heard. But in this scenario, I was a conduit for someone else's history and thoughts and feelings at a critical life juncture. I'd never had a muse like that before, and I wanted to do it again. I went straight back to the perfect person to inspire another song: Flavie. She demurred (*Why would anyone want to write a song about me?*) before agreeing to participate in an impromptu writing session. She was happy, she said, to see me looking like I was getting my act together.

Her exact words were, "It's about time."

For Flavie, exploring her history and creating a song took her back to the melancholy time when she was a single mom, filled with love for her daughters but facing the challenges of raising them alone. It took her back to being a spunky young woman who couldn't be told what to do or what kind of career was suitable for her. It harked back to her days on stage, singing and dancing in full costume and makeup, proud and happy. She giggled and sang and wiped away tears as she told me her story, and even though the song we ended up with was a simple melody with a two-chord chorus, it captured something enchanted for us both. At the end of our dialogue, we had the shape and sound for the aptly titled "Generous Heart."

I tinkered with the lyrics and music for a couple days, but the song had come together easily and well. Flavie and I sat side by side in an exam room and I sang it through, adding a few flourishes on the guitar, because it was, after all, for one of the most show-stopping people I'd ever met. A dancer through and through, she felt the music with her whole being, nodding her head and waving her graceful hands in time with the rhythm of her chorus:

> *You followed your dream*
> *Despite all the loss,*
> *Unstoppably you no matter the cost.*
> *Clearing my clouds*
> *While dancing your part,*
> *Shining your light*
> *With your generous heart.*

When we reached the end, she winked up at me and leaned her head against my shoulder.

"Thanks, Dr. E.," she said. "That's lovely."

Not wanting the moment to end, and knowing how much she loved Sinatra, I snapped my fingers and transitioned to a cheerful "Fly Me to the Moon." She picked it up instantly and gleefully, adding her thin but pitch-perfect voice to mine.

In the quiet moment at the end of the song, I watched her chest rise and fall, noting the labored breathing brought on by just a few minutes of engagement.

"Let's talk about how you're feeling," I said. "What can I do to make you more comfortable?"

"I don't want to talk about cancer right now," she said, shaking her head. "You know something? When I was a young widow, I thought my life was over."

I held out her water and she took a sip before continuing.

"But I'd hardly done anything yet. I had no idea how much was still ahead in the second act."

"You made the most of it, Flav," I said. "I mean, what a life!"

She smiled, wistful and bright-eyed.

"You're just starting your second act, too, Dr. E.," she said. "You've got work to do."

Humming the song on the way home, there was no question in my mind that the process we'd just been through was as healing as any treatment, medication, or intervention I'd been able to offer Flavie since we'd met.

It was a moment in time that did feel like the beginning of a new phase. Up until that year, I'd believed I had to separate my own personal church and state: music in one part of my life, medicine in the other. But none of it had been going very well. My saving grace was combining the two, honoring both parts of me. That simple choice put me on a path that felt consistent with my priorities, my passions, and my commitment to my patients.

The change was nothing less than life-changing, first because all the miserable physical symptoms I'd been suffering started to recede. I slept through one night, and then another, feeling fully rested for perhaps the first time since our move to California. I ate better and felt better, and my colitis went into remission. I started meditating, just a few minutes a day at first, and my migraines eased. My asthma—which had been managed in my childhood, eradicated in young adulthood, and raging in my first years of medical practice—retreated again, off to the remote corner of me it inhabits, where it stayed dormant. As a doctor I know how disheartening chronic interruptions to the basic routines of the body can be, and I was deeply grateful to reach a point where I could sleep, eat, pee, breathe, dream, and work out like a healthy person. As a result I felt strong and tuned in as a doctor, like I finally had enough to give.

♡

Ask anyone who works in advertising or the music industry and they can confirm that music sometimes works like a time machine. Dr. Oliver Sacks, the world-renowned neurologist and author of *The Man Who Mistook His Wife for a Hat*, wrote of a patient describing what he called an "intracranial jukebox." We all have one, filled with songs and tunes that ignite our minds, tapping into the sights, smells, tastes, tactile sensations, and emotions of moments they're eternally bound up with in our memories. Music, for reasons modern science still doesn't completely understand, transcends the normal bounds of brain activity. Advances in assessments like electroencephalograms and functional MRI prove that music touches and activates every corner of the human mind—even the evolutionarily primeval base of the brainstem. We're still figuring out the hows and whys, but we know for sure that our brains and music go *way* back, beyond the modern and even the ancient, to something prehistoric and elemental in the role of rhythm in human function.

Even though I wrote those first songs with patients for intuitive reasons, I started reading and researching about the power of music in medicine. I remembered well the logic of bringing arts to medicine from the humanities program at the Lombardi Cancer Center at Georgetown—how exercises, classes, and concerts forged bonds at all levels of interaction in the hospital. It had opened up previously nonexistent lines of communication. It had increased accurate reporting of symptoms and fostered more effective clinical responses. Since I'd been at Georgetown, research into the power of music in medicine had made giant leaps. Hundreds of studies indicated that music can ease pain, reduce stress, and boost immune function. It can soothe or it can energize. It can give strangers common ground and shared experiences. What's more, new research was finding that just as music can transport us to the past like it did for Flavie, it can also help us be more present and able to tap into the healthy, strong parts of ourselves. Music has the power to remind each of us of who we are, of our most positive facets and memories and capabilities.

Tapping into this power doesn't have to be as complicated or collaborative as writing a song with your oncologist (though that's an excellent way to go if it works for you!). My patients living with cancer tell me the simple, passive act of listening to music is the most effective way to lift or quiet their moods. Family members tell me music is magic, noting how it can create harmony where it might seem none could possibly be found. I always knew that to be true because I'd lived it when I was just a kid after my accident, unable to say a word but somehow fully expressive when I was singing. Even so, I continue to be amazed at the weight of its implications for my patients. If you are looking for a way to connect—patient to family, family to patient, or as a caregiver—there is little you can do wrong. If you want a starting place, there are a few easy ones anyone can use.

The first is the easiest. Set aside a little time every day to bask (or wallow, if the mood suits) in music you love. Play a song that brings back a treasured memory. Use music as an audible escape hatch and allow it to transport you to the past or the future or an alternate present that feels right. I've had patients who "conduct" orchestras blaring in their headphones, patients who get their rage out blasting Metallica, and patients who snuggle up with their partners for a few minutes every day to listen to music from weddings and parties and concerts they've seen together. The important thing isn't the soundtrack you choose; it's giving yourself over to it for a while, giving your emotions a healthy, restorative way out.

Music can help ease transitions too. Whether you need a little boost to get started in the morning, something to calm your nerves before or during a treatment, or a lullaby at night, choose a soundtrack of a few songs that fit the mood you're after. Research shows that if you routinely pair a particular playlist with an activity or time of day, that music can help you more easily and readily switch gears.

Music can also serve as a gateway to one of the most effective stress-relieving tools in the human toolbox: meditation. It is the one mind-body practice I can tell you with absolute authority works, because I do it every day, because my patients do it as often as they can, because it has changed our lives, bringing us gently back to the most centered, sane, peaceful versions of ourselves again and again.

When someone says *Just relax,* do you respond with *Are you joking?* It's hard to begin, to carve out 20 minutes, to let go of every nagging thing. When I started meditating, I did it in my car—the only place I felt comfortable isolating myself from interruption and distraction for 20 whole minutes.

It can be even more challenging to carve out time and focus when you're suffering from chemo brain, from depression, or from anxiety. Music can be the means to that end. A soft, steady instrumental track helps you breathe steadily, deeply, and slowly. It serves as a tool to help deflect the thoughts that inevitably come rushing in when we first slow down and try to quiet our minds. It's a place you can release those thoughts, acknowledging the worries and the urgencies with a simple, *Thanks, maybe later. Right now I'm just listening, just being.* In this context music serves as a synonym for the right now: this moment, this sound— experiences in which we can immerse ourselves and let every other thing go.

Turn on your music and turn down your raging thoughts for 20 minutes every day. Consider it a prescription.

CHAPTER 15

THE
OPEN ROAD

The grass isn't greener over there.
It's grass.
I'm here.
I'm here now.
Let's be here now and love it.

— *DAILY DOSE*, SEPTEMBER 2, 2019

In June of 2020, Caitlin Flanagan of *The Atlantic* wrote a column called "I Thought Stage IV Cancer Was Bad Enough" about being medically fragile during a pandemic (and so much more). The title grabbed me, and her eloquent voice arrested my attention as she disclosed one of the bittersweet truths about chronic and even terminal illness: life goes on.

When she first learned she had cancer, Flanagan wrote, a friend told her life would still move forward, that even when she was sick and in treatment she'd be in the thick of it. Of course she doubted.

Upon learning they have cancer, many patients think, *This is the end*. It's a natural response to earth-shaking news. But it's not true. In treatment, sickness, recovery, remission, and even decline—through all of it, life carries on. You laugh, cry, and love your people. Someone who's been there will tell you this not long after your diagnosis, perhaps promising good days and bad days. You may not believe them, but time always brings truth.

Years into treatment, Flanagan wrote, she opened her photo albums, expecting to see sad children or a mourning family, and instead found pictures of happy kids, family trips, school events. Turning the pages, she said, she realized she was looking at her life's work.

Flanagan's recognition of the love she'd shared and the work she'd done as a mother speaks to a universal and critical query: *If we know our time is finite, what do we do today? What do we choose as our life's work?*

I think about this nearly every day. The average American life span is in the ballpark of 78 years. That's 28,470 days; 683,000 hours; more than 40 million minutes. So much time to use or to waste, to show love or to be indifferent, to do something meaningful . . . or not.

But who among us is average? What if I only have a few years, or a few months, or a few days? When a third or half or all but one of these units of time is gone, will I look at the photo albums on my iCloud and think, *I'm glad. I loved. I lived.*

If I do, I'll have a lot of people who first came into my life as patients to thank on the other side—patients who allowed me to do life-affirming work, who pushed me to be better, who let me into their lives when they were taking stock of their life's work.

♡

Roger was the first patient who came to me in part because I was doing something a little different, coloring ever so slightly outside the lines of oncology. But instead of just noting or observing, he launched a reeling, rollicking melody that drew me further out.

He was a renaissance man—a mechanical savant, a musician, a traveler, a thinker, a person of integrity and action. He'd retired early to devote an act of his life to music—playing it, hearing it, and living it. He played the guitar and his wife, Gretchen, played the fiddle, and together they set out in an RV with bold intentions to make a folk music trek from sea to shining sea. Every morning, with another concert in the rearview mirror, Roger would tumble out of his camper, look at the landscape, and think about his good fortune. He and the love of his life were doing what they wanted, when they wanted, how they wanted. They were side by side on top of the world.

They made their way from Southern California across the country and then up the coast. By New York, Roger had a backache that wouldn't quit. By Connecticut, he had the nagging sense that it was a new kind of trouble. By Massachusetts, plagued by pain that wouldn't subside with medicine or rest, ice or heat, he made a detour to an emergency room.

It only took an X-ray for the doctor to gently suggest to Roger that it was time to go home. There appeared to be cancer in his bones. He should get off the road and find a specialist.

Three thousand miles later, the musicians were back in San Diego. A member of the local music community, Roger had somehow heard about the song I wrote for Chuck, and despondent as he was the first time we met, he told me that even in cancer treatment, he wanted music in his life.

Just weeks after spine surgery, he embarked on a chemo regimen to push back against the multiple myeloma inhabiting his bone marrow. Because of the damage done before his diagnosis, Roger wore a bulky, constricting brace to support his back, and he moved with the slow, deliberate caution of a man who was hurting.

Still, this stout and balding fellow with a tidy grey beard and wide expressive eyes was radiant. He was Santa Claus meets Paul Simon, exuding positivity, intelligence, and creative spirit. In the treatment room, his warm presence drew everyone in.

I saw a great deal of Roger in the first months of his care because he came in for blood work and treatment every week. At first his movement was limited by the brace, but as weeks and months passed, he mastered it, saying it was becoming just another part of him—not his favorite, but something he was figuring out how to live with. As his treatment progressed, in addition to monitoring his body's response, I asked about his music. He was the real deal—a guitarist who could play in any style—but his favorite was the gentle energy of folk music. "You should have seen us on the road," he said, reminding me that Gretchen was an accomplished musician in her own right. "Maybe one day we'll play for you."

I told him I couldn't wait and joked that I might recruit him into my one-man therapy-room band. That was the moment our relationship changed. I would still be his doctor for years to come, but I was about to become his fan, his friend, and, from time to time, his student.

Roger's treatments took an hour, but many patients were in the chemo room for longer stretches of time—spending several hours tethered to IVs that delivered harsh medications as slowly as possible so as not to shock or damage their systems. As soon as he was strong enough to sit tall and hold his guitar, Roger and Gretchen started showing up for his infusions with instrument cases in hand. After his infusion, instead of going home to rest like most patients want and need to do, Roger would pick up his guitar and Gretchen would settle her fiddle on her shoulder, and they'd play for

the room. I'd been offering up ditties and even a few personal ballads, but this was something else. Roger strummed
and picked with precision. Gretchen's fingers flew and her
bow seemed to take on a life of its own as she played individual notes and raucous chords in the same stroke. Their
melodies lilted and raced, swung high and low, and lifted
every patient, family member, nurse, and doctor who heard
them. We'd come out of our offices and migrate down the
hall, tapping and dancing and humming our way closer to
this couple who somehow changed the entire ambiance of
the place with their presence.

A few times I tried to join in, but Roger was a better
instrumentalist than I. It was more fun to watch, and more
rewarding to catch him as he was packing up his guitar and
ask his advice. He never failed to patiently show me how to
tackle a difficult riff or pick out a challenging chord.

Roger endured months of difficult treatment, but when
it was over, he was in remission. He and Gretchen started
talking about going back on the road, but it wasn't meant to
be. Gretchen, who had been kind and funny, devoted and
patient throughout Roger's treatment, suffered a stroke and
started down a long road to her own recovery. The couple
sold their RV and moved into an assisted living complex. I
was heartbroken for these friends who had come to be such
an important part of my life—right up until the next time I
saw them together. I'd been prepared to share in their sense
of loss for the dream that had come to an end and hear
about the challenges of the months they'd been MIA from
my life. Instead they started talking about their new community with the kind of enthusiasm I'd heard when they
shared their adventures in the Badlands, the Smokies, and
the Adirondack Park.

"You should see these walking trails," they told me during one visit. "They're gorgeous. The trees are all in bloom." On another they reported having discovered the vast kitchen in the complex and all its wonders. They made new friends, learned new games, and held hands in my office like teenagers. Roger entered a five-year remission but continued to stop by to play music for patients in the treatment room.

Even as the paths available to them narrowed, they continued exploring together.

Roger taught me to be a better musician. He also taught me to be a better person. His willingness to embrace the positive in even the most disheartening circumstances is something I continue to carry with me. The way he shared music with the rest of my patients was an affirmation of everything I believed and hoped music could accomplish in oncology. When he and Gretchen played, they transformed the room into a different place, somewhere you might want to sit a while, a center of healing and community.

When Roger got sick again after outpacing every likely prognosis for his condition, he came back to that same room again as a patient. There were different people in the recliners, but the sense of their shared circumstances and what he had brought to the struggle hadn't changed. He still had kind eyes and a warm heart as he made friends with his chemo neighbors and encouraged them with tales of his long and productive remission.

One afternoon I sat with a group of patients and asked for their help. Many of them, like me, had gotten to know the man behind the guitar. Together we wrote a song for him and about him and called it "The Open Road."

A year later my friend was gone, his life's work a testament to his character and talent. He was a husband, a father, a careful and hard worker. He was a traveler, a singer, a guitar and banjo player. He was a volunteer and a loyal friend.

In the end he had 74 years. That's about 27,000 days. 648,000 hours. More than 38 million minutes of life in this world.

I like to think that in his afterlife, a big RV was waiting for Roger, and an entire universe that's his to explore.

CHAPTER 16

SPOONFUL

You're leaving a legacy every moment.
Every moment you show up matters.

— *Daily Dose*, March 1, 2020

If you ask American adults what action most allows them to feel their freedom, many will tell you it is driving. That's why teenagers covet and pursue it above all other goals; why seniors cling to their licenses when the kids and grandkids start dropping hints about giving them up. It's also a privilege people with debilitating and terminal illnesses work mightily to protect, because behind the wheel they are independent. Nobody wants to give that up.

One patient battling a deadly and inoperable brain tumor summed it up as she wistfully recounted her last day driving for me. "I only went a few miles," she said. "I let the dog ride shotgun and we got a milkshake. I was free as a bird."

For Roger, driving was an exquisite part of his journey—the long-awaited pleasures of having one concert behind and another ahead. For another patient who profoundly impacted my life, however, driving was an escape—an excuse to speed away from his troubles until he found a way to reframe his purpose.

♡

Ben was a big, boisterous retired CEO who came to me when he was already nearly out of medical options. He was an imposing guy with a gruff voice and a presence that couldn't be ignored. He was the kind of person everyone looks to for answers, and so he seemed oddly out of place in an exam room asking questions.

During our first visit, I asked him to tell me about his medical history, and he quickly diverted into business history instead, talking about his work as a CEO, moving from company to company, breathing new life into each one in turn. In his late 50s, he was at the peak of his impressive career—old enough to exude power, young enough to never be mistaken for a business-world has-been. He'd worked in Tokyo and Moscow, Paris and Beijing. It was his job, he said animatedly, to solve big companies' biggest problems and help them regain profitability.

"Until I got this damned cancer," he finished. Even as he said it, he deflated, slumping in his chair.

"Tell me what you've been through so far," I asked.

Ben recounted a year of surgeries and therapies in an increasingly exasperated tone. "Nobody wants to give me a straight answer," he said. "I ask a simple question, and I get a load of crap. I've researched this. I know where it's going. I just want two things at this point: truth and medication."

I got the sense that lung cancer might have been the first problem this man had run up against in his entire adult life that he couldn't solve. He was angry about it, cursing treatments that hadn't changed his prognosis and medications that made him feel worse instead of better. As someone who'd spent decades bending individuals and companies to his will, he didn't know how to handle being susceptible to something as evasive and all-consuming as disease.

Not surprisingly, I was not Ben's first oncologist. In fact, it appeared he'd already run through several, "firing" each in turn. He'd already exhausted the standard treatment protocols, and his clinical trial options were limited. His cancer had been beaten back multiple times, and the recurrence that brought him to me would be the one that would persist. I told him that because of the extent of his disease, my role would not be to try to save him from his cancer but to help him live with it. I would, I promised, give him only straight answers.

"Can you write me a script for medical pot?" he asked.

"I can."

"Good," he nodded. "I think I'd like that."

I certainly hoped I could offer Ben something more.

When I asked about his family and how they'd been coping with his illness, Ben's bluster faded again.

"I used to be on the road all the time," he said. "My wife would fly out and meet me sometimes for the weekend. We'd have a few days here and there at home together. Now I'm underfoot all the time. I'm not working. Before, even when I wasn't working, I was."

"Plus," he continued, "a lot of days I just feel like hell."

I asked if he liked to read or had hobbies he was enjoying at home, and he smiled and said conspiratorially, "I do have one thing. It's a car—a Beemer. God, I love it. I get behind the wheel and drive along the coast and it feels like a last gasp of freedom."

"Does your wife ride with you?" I asked.

"Not much," he shrugged. "I guess I should ask her."

I nodded, and he said, "Hey, do you want to see it? The car? It's a beauty."

Of course I wanted to see the car, but first we laid out a plan for Ben's care—one that included a newly approved chemo medication. Ben nodded in agreement at each suggestion, and after we got his prescriptions in order, he led me to the parking lot to see the gleaming racing convertible.

He opened the doors and invited me to sit inside. It was probably the nicest car I'd ever seen. He asked if I'd like to go for a ride. On any given day before my dance with Flavie, I'd have declined—thinking I had to maintain some vestige of propriety between doctor and patient. But that was before. I had one more patient to see, and Ben waited. Afterward I grabbed my keys and jacket and we practically raced out the door, like kids skipping school. We put the top down and headed for the highway. I was exhilarated and Ben grinned—a transformation from the man who'd glowered and grimaced in the exam room.

As we drove he blasted a Muddy Waters CD and sang along. For the next half hour, we were just a couple guys driving to the blues.

When we stopped for coffee, Ben spoke about his wife and daughter, and about how much he felt at a loss to help them through his illness. When I pointed out that his inability to control or erase the single greatest medical scourge of humankind wasn't something he should beat himself up about, he voiced what hundreds of thousands of men, women, and children who've had cancer have felt before him.

"It's my body," he said. "How can I be so powerless?"

After that Ben scheduled his appointments for the end of my day, and our rides became regular adventures. Over the months he was my patient, I encouraged him to get closer to his family rather than continue to pull away, and one day as we drove, he started talking about how beautiful it was on the patio at his house. It was the first time he'd shared any detail about his home. He'd never noticed before, he said, but lately he and the family had been sitting out there mornings. He talked about going with his wife to the farmer's market and about finally taking her along on one of his joyrides—how she'd worn a scarf over her hair like a movie star and laughed as she stretched her arms up through the open top, pretending to catch the wind in her hands.

In the beginning Ben offered me a lot of advice, about running my practice, about investing, about real estate. I think he just wanted to share some of his hard-earned knowledge. As our time together went on, though, the nature of his advice started to change, focusing more on family and legacy and less on success and prosperity.

"It's a little late for me to be figuring this out," he told me one day, "but I've spent most of my life chasing after big moments—takeovers and launches and deals. I blew by all the little bullshit stuff of life—how I slept and what I ate and what it feels like to sit beside somebody who knows and loves you with a glass of wine and the radio on.

"I'm looking at it all now," he continued, "and I think I miscalculated. That bullshit—the day-to-day stuff that feels like nothing in between the big moments—that's the beauty. I almost missed it."

That afternoon, he blared Howlin' Wolf's "Spoonful" as we drove along the coast with the top down.

"I'm telling you, Doc," he said, rolling his head to the music, the hard edge I'd seen in him at the beginning of our partnership gone. "The bullshit is the beauty."

♡

The lesson Ben was learning in this too-short second chance with his family was one I knew I needed to take to heart in my own life. One of the most daunting things about oncology is that you never really detach from it. You can't wash your hands of soul work when you come home at night—not the celebrations and not the mourning. You know your patients are on the other side of the equation, and they certainly can't shut it down at will. Cancer doesn't work that way for anyone. The profession's weight and emotion permeate the fabric of your being whether you're at the office, the hospital, on call, taking your kids to the zoo, or on a date with your spouse. When an ER attending calls and says she has a patient with "breast cancer everywhere," when a new headache turns out to be metastatic disease from a distant organ, when every person who crosses into your exam room is somebody's mother, father, sister, brother, daughter, or son in some form of peril, there's no mistaking the gravity of the work.

My patients are a treasured part of my life. Separating that piece of me from the part that is husband, father, son, brother, and friend is impossible. That makes it far too easy to check out instead of staying present while I'm having sandwiches with my family or washing dishes next to my wife, teaching my daughter to drive or helping my son with his homework. After spending time with Ben, though, I could almost hear his voice in my head when I'd start to drift away from my family. *If you're not careful, you'll miss it,* he said.

My amazing wife had, of course, been telling me this all along. Sometimes she'd look at me or touch my hand with hers and say, *Be here right now.* She'd bring me back. Ben made me mindful of the business-as-usual stuff I was tuning out—conversations and events Julie might not find worth the trouble of reminding me to check in on.

There are few things sadder or more frustrating than a revelation that comes too late. I was lucky. My kids were still small and my wife was still loving and patient when Ben came into my life and showed me how hard it is to make up for lost time. The mantra he inspired—one I share with family, friends, patients, and anyone else who will listen—is *Start now.* Whatever it is you want to make happen, do it a little bit today. Eat a vegetable. Take a walk. Kiss your spouse. Turn off your phone. Write how you feel. Sing. Dance. Pray.

Do something fun. Do something kind. Talk with your kids. Call your mom.

Even the smallest actions we take have consequences, and the actions we take repeatedly become habits and lifestyles and part of who we are. If you're living, dying, busy, or bored—do one small thing that makes you feel better. Then do another.

CHAPTER 17

TRIPLE CROWN

Your trillion cells put up a fight.
A ray of sun to end the night.
Can't keep you down,
Won't let you down,
My triple crown.

— SONG FOR VIVIAN, 2020

One of the first and toughest challenges of medical school is coming face-to-face with death in the anatomy lab in the form of a research cadaver. Death is a looming presence throughout any medical career, but its incarnation in this form is a difficult and draining rite of passage. As a 22-year-old med student, my first impression as I walked into the cavernous, cold lab and saw each research station with its neatly wrapped body was a wave of wonder that I had somehow gotten there as one of the living rather than one of the dead. From time to time, something I'd seen or heard reminded me of my near-fatal bike accident, but standing in the lab, my senses were overwhelmed not with what I was observing in the room, but with what I'd felt nearly a decade earlier—the taste of blood in my mouth; the woozy blur of fading in and out of consciousness; the cognizance that my leg was bent at an unnatural angle; the pain that was so complete my entire body was enveloped in it.

Yet there I was, tall and skinny, warm and alive. And on my lab table was someone who had gone the other way.

It was with shaky hands that I unwrapped the body assigned to me. I had never seen a dead person before, much less touched one. Death had been an abstract notion in my life, but here I was, on the cusp of violating the human vessel in the name of clinical science. I didn't know how to separate body and soul. It was too sacred.

My specimen was a female in her 70s, and she wore pink nail polish that reminded me of my grandmother's hands. I called her Molly. What I wanted to do that first day was grieve for her and betray my complete unsuitability to practice medicine, but I was too proud to let that happen.

Instead I reminded myself again and again, that day and every lab day after, that Molly had donated her body for a purpose, that she had chosen to be an instrument of learning. It was only when I took that assumption to the next level that I could do any worthwhile work. I imagined that I, personally, had her blessing, that her soul was somehow in the room, gently encouraging me to learn from her. *I honor your soul* became a mental and sometimes spoken mantra to get me through as I studied her body. *Thank you. I honor your soul.* I committed the lessons of the lab deep in my memory, swearing I would use everything Molly taught me to one day heal and help patients.

I'd been a class clown for my whole life up until then (and was frequently one after), but the sanctity of that process was a jarring wake-up call about what we were getting into.

In practice now, going on 30 years later, I still think of Molly and her sacrifice. I think of her when I read the results of a PET scan and can visualize what's happening inside the liver or lung, kidney or bones of a person who is very much alive. I think of her in moments when I have to consider the limits of what the human body can endure. And I think of her most when I can tell a patient that, thanks to insights gained through screening and testing, we've found something early and small and treatable.

Yes, it's there is the hardest part to share. We see this mass or node or spot that looks like trouble. It looks enough like cancer that we need to figure it out.

It helps to be able to also say that because the patient asked for screening, or because their friend or mother or doctor recommended it and they showed up, we're in a strong position to manage what comes next.

Life in oncology is full of stories of cancer caught just in time, but they're often overshadowed by the ones about times it was found too late. Thanks in large part to routine mammograms, more than 60 percent of breast cancers in the U.S. are found at stage I. Thanks to regular Pap smears, the incidence of cervical cancer has dropped by half since the 1970s. Colorectal cancer screening has steadily reduced the rate of colon cancer in adults over 50 for the past two decades. On the horizon, we're looking forward to ever more sophisticated and predictive screening tools—like a blood biomarker test sensitive to genetic hints of disease years before measurable tumors develop, and genetic screening that will provide a more complete and complex picture of each person's unique predispositions to disease than we are capable of deciphering today.

Early detection is the best treatment—the one with the most promise for positive outcomes and the one that spares patients more invasive and uncomfortable interventions than anything else. Each year thousands of patients undergo treatment and then get on with their lives because testing exposed a lurking threat. The privilege of telling even one person *You are going to be all right* after an incidence of cancer is nothing less than life-affirming. The fact is, this is something most oncologists get to do often, delivering good news and sending a new veteran to join the nearly 17 million cancer survivors in the U.S. alone at this writing.

From time to time, I get to have this conversation with the same patient twice. The incidence of multiple primary cancers is not uncommon, but the patient who faces a fresh diagnosis time and again (and again and again) is rare—even when she's had nine decades to experience them.

♡

Some people have all the luck, or not much of it, depending on your point of view. Ten years ago, a patient came into my office and in doing so swept me up on her journey as a living example of both. Vivian is a 90-year-old four-time cancer survivor. Hers were not four battles against a single disease, but wars against four different ones. She's had breast, colon, skin, and lung cancers, and she's beaten them all.

I don't like to frame medical stories in terms of "winning" or "losing" against cancer. It's not always a healthy perspective when you're coping with disease, and the interplay between people and illness and their lives before, during, and after is never quite that simple. But Vivian is indomitable, and there's no way to tell her story without making an exception and admitting that, yes, she did kick cancer's ass.

She was a spry 81, with square-rimmed glasses and short grey hair, when we first met. Her diagnosis was malignant neoplasm of the colon. Vivian told me, almost offhandedly, that she'd had cancer before—breast cancer in her 60s that had been effectively treated and hadn't come back.

When a cancer that originates in one part of the body arises in another, it's made of the same kind of cells as the original, and still identified as such. Breast cancer is still breast cancer, for example, even if it develops in the liver or lungs. Vivian's new diagnosis didn't fall into this category.

Her new tumor type was distinct from the one she'd experienced before.

Unfortunately the colon cancer hadn't stayed put. A single positive lymph node, discovered during her surgical resection, raised the stakes by making it a stage III disease. A colleague of mine sums up this stage by saying it means "the horses are out of the barn." The implication of that ominous metaphor is that we're dealing with Cancer Gone Wild, that it's rampaging along and we might be powerless to catch it.

Experience has taught me to take a different view: *hold your horses.* Even though nearby spread of any malignancy is a more complex problem than cancer that can be eliminated at its origin, this is not a too-late scenario. More than half of patients diagnosed with stage III colon cancer (defined by regional but not distant spread) are still alive five years on. For those who have only a single lymph node impacted, the odds are better. Vivian's affected lymph node meant there was more work to do, but I was able to tell her that I see patients every day who are successfully pushing back on stage III spread.

That was the headline.

The rest of the story was that surgery alone would not be enough to fully eradicate a cancer that had invaded nearby structures. Research tells us that even when we cut out cancer that's spread, microscopic malignant cells remain. To have realistic hope for a long-term cure, Vivian's next step would be a chemotherapy regimen strong enough to root out those lingering cells. It was adjuvant therapy—treatment given after the primary intervention (in this case, surgery) to lower the risk of recurrence. To complicate matters, the gold standard of treatment for Vivian's case was also one of the worst-tolerated chemotherapy regimens I prescribe.

I was a little afraid to give it to her. Part of my job is considering whether a patient is strong enough to get through treatment. I always lay out all options, but if you ask, *What do you think I should do?* or *Would you do it?*, or the highest litmus test, *Would you recommend this for YOUR mom?*, the only acceptable answer is an honest one. Would I undergo this treatment myself? In a heartbeat. Would I ask my own grandma to do it? Probably?

Sizing up a standoff between sweet Vivian and this daunting regimen, any sane person would worry.

So we sat down and we talked about it—about the treatment and what it might mean for her to have it at an age when some patients experience severe side effects and take longer than average to recover from them. We talked about the fact that it would take time—several months—to get through the process, and that some patients become too sick to complete the full regimen. We talked about the breast cancer she'd had before we met and how it had been caught early and treated conservatively, leaving more options in the future-treatment toolbox. We talked about whether there were any other health considerations that might weigh on her choice.

The facts were all out, and it was time for me to ask what she was thinking, what her priorities were, what else I could do to help her make an informed decision.

I had just read a study that examined adjuvant chemotherapy in colon cancer patients in terms of who takes it and who opts out. The data showed that the older a patient is, the less likely he or she is to participate. The trend wasn't surprising, but the actual numbers were still a shock: 92 percent of patients under 65 received the treatment. So did a wide majority of patients 65–80. After 80, the number of patients accepting adjuvant chemo plummeted to 27 percent.

There are plenty of reasons for an age-related discrepancy in accepting treatment: focus on quality of life over quantity; the financial and physical costs of treatment; logistical challenges of appointments and follow-ups; incomplete recovery from tumor resection; existing conditions that might reduce efficacy or add to suffering. Also, the study's authors postulated, doctors might sometimes recommend less than the accepted standard of care because they, like me, are a little afraid.

I waited for Vivian's input, mentally mapping out what we'd do next if she did opt for adjuvant treatment and if she did not.

She didn't keep me in suspense for long.

"When do you think we can get started?" she asked.

It was only then, when I felt my shoulders and back unknot, that I realized this was what I hoped she'd choose. Deep down, I believed she was up to it.

A week later Vivian was in the treatment room for round one. As with many chemo "cocktails," a component of the solution slowly dripping through into her veins was cyto-toxic—destructive to all cells, not just the bad ones. I'm certain I speak for everyone in my field when I say that I can't wait for the day when toxic-to-the-whole-body chemo-therapies are a thing we remember from medicine's past. In my lifetime we've made significant strides in being able to mitigate the side effects of these treatments, but we have a long way to go in figuring out how to make them less toxic to healthy cells. Vivian's treatment would make her tired and nauseous. It would make her vulnerable to infection. It might thin her hair or cause sores in her mouth. It would also subject her to the strange side effect of hypersensitivity to cold. Cold drinks, cold floors, cold bannisters, cold air—all of them were about to become intolerable.

We'd talked about the possibilities, and she'd come pre-pared. She was dressed in soft, warm layers, with a pair of mittens in her lap and a room-temperature bottle of green tea on her table.

She was reading quietly, and when I stopped to check on her progress, I casually asked what her book was about.

She gave me a mischievous grin and flipped it over so I could see the cover.

Bad Days in History: A Gleefully Grim Chronicle of Misfortune, Mayhem, and Misery for Every Day of the Year

I laughed out loud.

"Really, Viv? Of all the books?"

"Keeps things in perspective," she said. Then she sipped her tea, patted her mittens, flipped the book back over and resumed reading.

"I'll give this to you when I finish!" she called after me as I made my way out of the room.

With the strength of someone half her age and a willfulness that was timeless, Vivian got through the full course of her treatment, riding the waves of chemo-induced discomfort one after another.

And then it was gone. Her scans were clear, and she was cancer free again.

♡

After Vivian's chemo, I saw her every three months, then every six months—always hoping for her continued good health but managing her screening with a close eye. With the exception of a squamous cell skin carcinoma—caught early and removed completely—she was amazingly healthy, rolling through her 80s in style.

With another cancer journey in the rearview mirror, we had time to chat a little about our taste in books and our shared love of music. She'd done some acting, she told me, and some singing and dancing, and she'd played the piano.

Of course she did. It was cancer that brought us together, but this was fertile common ground. We laughed about everything from our shared experiences with childhood piano lessons to her decades-long song-and-dance partnership with her husband, Jack.

One day she brought in a playbill featuring two caricatures: on one side, a dashing man swinging a cane and doffing a top hat, on the other, a woman in a flapper dress standing beside a piano, her skirt and beaded necklace captured mid-swing. When I looked closer at the flapper's jawline, her wide-set mouth, her square-rimmed glasses, it was unmistakably Vivian. The cover read, *Shades of Vaudeville*. I marveled at the surprises she kept bringing—always keeping me on my toes.

At the six-year mark, something was amiss with Vivian's blood work. Since she was a colon cancer survivor, we followed her tumor marker level—staying vigilant for hints of trouble. When her labs showed an elevation, I thought, *There it is again, damn it.* A PET scan revealed a lung nodule. It wasn't big, but it didn't belong. There were not a lot of explanations that would end well for my patient. Colon cancer metastatic to the lung would mean a stage IV recurrence. It would be treatable but not curable, and it would likely be more resistant to intervention than anything Vivian had already overcome.

I worried. She worried. She got a biopsy and we waited.

Occasionally in the world of cancer treatment, just like in every other aspect of our lives, God winks. Things are not as they seem. I braced myself for Vivian's biopsy to prove her colon cancer had spread, weighing what an 88-year-old woman with multiple previous cancers could handle—no matter how much of a pistol she happened to be.

The biopsy didn't come back stage IV anything. It was a brand-new cancer, this time of the lung. It was stage I, caught just as it started to take root, and curable with radiation alone. Vivian got through that just like she'd gotten through everything else, and as I write this she is, once again, cancer free.

Vivian and I wrote a song together called "Triple Crown," a nod to the three big, bad cancers she's overcome. But there's another, different triple crown at play here. It doesn't make for any lilting lyrics, but in my world its components are beautiful anyway. Mammogram. Colonoscopy. Post-treatment tumor marker readings. Are you up to date? Say yes and it will be music to my ears.

CHAPTER 18

THE MESSAGE

What we need right now is CPR:
Connection. Presence. Resilience.

— *Daily Dose*, July 18, 2018

Hope's case is the kind that makes oncologists want to curl up and cry—a young mother, with almost no risk factors, fine one day and diagnosed with stage IV breast cancer the next. She came to my office on a December morning with a PET scan that showed metastatic disease in her liver and her bones. With bright eyes, delicate features, and a sprinkling of freckles across the bridge of her nose, she looked even younger than her 36 years. She was so distraught she could hardly speak, and when she did it was to say she couldn't believe the Christmas right around the corner was going to be her last. Her husband said he kept coming back to the unfairness of it, of cancer striking a woman who was kind to her core.

"She's the most loving mother," Paul said. "She brings home strays. She fosters dogs and cats. And birds! She takes care of everyone."

There are times when all I have for patients is news that's hard to hear, when I have to scavenge among harsh facts for every glimmer of hope. Sometimes that hope is relief from discomfort; sometimes it's directness where honesty has been lacking; sometimes it's news of a drug or trial or procedure that might brighten a patient's prospects for the near or long term. But sometimes I get to say that I've seen the particular phantom the patient is grappling with defeated. That first day I told Hope that despite the red alert of her scan, I'd seen the kind of cancer she was dealing with respond to treatment in the past. I believed she had a chance to achieve remission.

She had a hard time trusting that. The words *stage IV* weighed on her, hung in the room. I took her hands in mine and said, "You remind me of my little sister, so that's how I'm going to treat you, okay?"

She nodded.

"The next few months are going to be awful. You're going to feel worse before you feel better. Chemotherapy is hard core. We can reasonably hope that it will scrub this cancer out of your bones and give you time. I wish I could tell you how much, but there's no way to know. Right now, I just need you to give me a chance. Let's fight it. We'll do it together."

In the months that followed, I saw Hope frequently and sometimes sat with her in the chemo room, chatting with her and Paul. I asked how they met, and she told me he'd lived in the apartment above hers, that he thought she was cute but didn't have the nerve to ask her out. Then one day she was out watering the plants on her balcony and he lowered a note on a fishing line, asking her to dinner.

I complimented Paul on his creative approach, and he smiled, winked, and said, "Can't argue with success!"

As her chemo progressed, Hope got sicker, to the point that there were times she thought she was dying. I gave her my cell number and told her to call anytime. We texted often, me encouraging her to push through, to focus on everything she had to fight for. One afternoon when she called, I told her about my bike accident and how my dad had told me not to take my life for granted.

"I think about that every day," I said, "and I think about patients like you who've been told *You're stage IV* and had to process everything that's implied with that. People like us are in on a big secret: that every day is a brand-new second chance—and that it might just be the last one. We have to try not to waste any of them."

Hope was trying. I knew she was, and I also knew it was increasingly difficult for her to appreciate her days when so many of them were filled with pain and nausea and worry about her family.

Then one day it was Paul who called. He told me he was losing her. Even though Hope had finished her grueling chemo regimen, she was still sick from it, and she was sinking so deep into depression, he was afraid there wasn't going to be any way to get her back. She was talking about dying, sleeping all the time, crying when she was awake.

"I can't break her out of it," he said. "It's like she's already left me."

I had used every bit of positivity I could summon, every medication, every trick and suggestion I had to give, but Hope was spiraling, and now her husband, steadfast and supportive throughout her ordeal, needed something else. With every medical intervention already underway, I offered the one thing I still hadn't attempted to do for Hope—the outlier that wasn't a treatment but that might be able to connect with her on a level nothing else seemed to reach.

"We could write her a song," I said. "We can use it to remind her what she's about. We could do it together."

That day Paul and I stayed on the phone, talking about lyrics along with Hope's upcoming tests and appointments. We came up with lines about him asking her to dinner, about how much love and comfort she gave others, about the future they still had. He told me how she'd wipe their daughters' eyes when either of them cried, kiss their cheeks, and tell them everything would be okay—how he wished it could be that easy to console the love of his life. We called the song "The Message." Paul's a musician, so we decided to play it together.

Hope's next appointment was cause for celebration. Her first scan after finishing chemo came back negative, the cancer that shadowed her bones and organs months earlier gone. I had hoped to see joy in her face when she heard the news, but she was withdrawn and quiet. So we tried a different tack. Paul went to get his djembe drum from his car. When I walked Hope into the empty chemo room and picked up my guitar, he was waiting. We told her we'd written a song for her, that we wanted to remind her how much her love means to everyone in her life. I have played hundreds of songs in my life and I've often played for strangers, but that day my hands shook. There was so much more at stake than the notes or the lyrics, the performance or the sound. The woman looking from me to her husband and back again had been trudging closer and closer to a precipice for months. She'd peered over the edge, and ever since, she'd struggled to turn back to the people who loved her. Medically Hope was as free as she could ever expect to be again in her life. Her scan report said NED: no evidence of disease. We should have been celebrating, but the moment had rung hollow. Paul had said she'd already left him.

We were going to do this one last crazy thing to try to bring her back.

When I glanced over at Paul so we could start in unison, he was searching his wife's face, anxious and hopeful.

I strummed the guitar and started to sing the first verse:

> *A message on a fishing pole,*
> *A message that you're always whole.*

A message of hope,
Never give up, nope,
On the message.

Hope's eyes widened and she leaned in.

What you take is what you give,
It's the message of how you live.
Take in a stray,
Each and every day,
It's your message.

Paul shifted the rhythm of the drums, moving toward the chorus, and I matched his tempo with the guitar.

Hope will appear,
Wash away the tears;
Hope will appear,
We'll be together, my dear . . .

When I looked at Hope again, her eyes were shining with tears and she had both hands covering her mouth. We sang her song, shaky at first and then stronger, belting out the chorus. Finally we waited, silent, for her response.

Hope jumped up and threw her arms around Paul, then hugged me. She showed more animation and joy in that moment than we'd seen from her in weeks.

"I can't believe you wrote that," she said. "It's one of the nicest things anyone's ever done for me."

Hope accepted her song and embraced it like a talisman, a touchstone in her ongoing battle against the phantom. At this writing she remains in remission. She is raising her daughters and fostering her dogs, laughing and singing and continuing to engage her fears. When she starts worrying about the future, she calls and we talk about living and dying. We talk about the fact that whether you've been stricken with cancer or mowed down by a station wagon, the experience of being knocked flat and coming nose to nose with death has to be a call to live.

♡

Moments of depression and anxiety are inevitable in oncology on all sides of the equation; patients and families (especially day-to-day caregivers) and health professionals all get beaten down by the changes cancer brings to our lives. For people who've suffered clinical depression in their pre-cancer lives, disease can be an especially powerful catalyst for a new bout with an old nemesis.

Everyone dealing with a cancer diagnosis experiences moments of sadness and fear—healthy responses to horrible, no good, very bad news. But for many of us, it's more than that. It can bring you to the point where you don't want to get out of bed, or eat, or connect with the people who love you.

For caregivers things are hard in a different way. Nearly half deal with depression and anxiety as they stand in the shadows, schlep coats and lists of medications, hold hands and pat backs, and wait, wait, wait.

Among doctors, burnout and depression are rife. In an anonymous survey, 90 percent said they'd been depressed but only a third had asked for help. It can be a unique burden for the person whose life's work is healing others to admit that he or she needs help healing too. I have been there, and I owe my emotional and physical recovery to patients like Flavie and Chuck and Roger. They showed me that instead of taking a step back, like so many physicians instinctively do when they reach a point where they feel they can't help, I can get closer and foster healing in another way. That change shifted my perception of my work. Instead of it draining me, it became life-affirming. It made me recognize the privilege in being able to actually help somebody every day. Pandemic me has gotten pretty fierce about this, more focused on finding a way to make a difference. My mind often jumps back to the Rolling Stones' "You Can't Always Get What You Want." What I *want* is to wave a magic wand and cure cancer. *Abracadabra* and that's it. Until that becomes technologically possible, though, I'm pursuing smaller, more grown-up wants. I want to sit down with one patient at a time, to listen with both ears and with my heart, to figure out something I can do to make things a little better right now.

As a patient or a caregiver, you'd be equally well-served by focusing on what you can do today.

Today I can take my pills even though I despise them.

Today I can eat something a little more nourishing than what I ate yesterday.

Today I can call my doctor to talk about the symptom that's been bothering me, the one I don't want to talk about—because that's what my doctor is there for.

Today when I look at the person I love who's been hurting, I can do something loving. We'll bake a cake, or take a walk, or snuggle up and watch a movie.

Today I can use my phone—as a phone. I can utilize its power for connecting with another human being instead of letting apps add to my intellectual and emotional overload.

What else helps? Be honest about how you feel and what you need, and ask the people you love to do the same. The oncology office becomes a quasi-couples counseling center more often than you'd imagine, simply because it's a place where families have to talk about things that have been going unsaid. A friend of mine who lived with breast cancer for nearly a decade told me saying the things that were hurting and frightening her out loud helped her find a way to live with them. "The more I told people and spread it out," she explained, "the less I was carrying."

When you get frustrated, don't feel bad about it. Have some self-compassion. Of course you have fears. Of course you are angry. It is *not* fair. Take a little time every day to give those feelings their moment. When your pain or fear is tightening its grip, take a few minutes to hear it—a brief audience for your mad, manic, or morose side. Listen without judgment and then let those thoughts go. Imagine blowing them away like dandelion fuzz—out of your head, out of the room, out of your life. Do it with a deep breath so you push them fast and far.

I tell my patients that *hope* stands for *hold on, pain ends*. When you discover for yourself that this is true, pass it on. It takes a special kind of bravery to share the struggle of your life with strangers, but it offers a special kind of healing in return. Hope has done it, opening her generous heart to other patients who are new to the experience and scared. She tells them that if she can fight her way back from the brink of utter darkness to embrace her partner and her children, they can come back too.

If none of this is working, if you're overwhelmed, ask for help—as much as you need. Your struggle is the reason friendships and counseling and support groups exist. No matter what you're going through, there is someone farther down the road who would like to hold your hand, answer your questions, reassure you there are good days to come. There is also someone out there who's devoted a lifetime to helping patients and families work through their frustrations and grief who wants to be there for you. They can do it in person, or on the phone, or over Zoom. If you don't know where to find a connection, ask your oncologist. Connecting patients to support resources is part of what we do. Find a way to share your pain so you don't have to carry it all yourself.

CHAPTER 19

I AM THE WARRIOR

That moment?
The end of the world as you know it.
A new now already in the works.
You have power still,
The power to create now,
And now,
And even now.

— *DAILY DOSE*, JUNE 28, 2019

Even after all these years in California, deep down I still see myself as a son of Philadelphia. For a long time, I identified most strongly with the broken, skinny kid who left the hospital at 13 years old, a different person than I'd been when I arrived. But on my good days, my best days, I like to think I have a streak of another Philly guy going on—just a little bit of Rocky.

It's there when I work out, and when I run up a couple steps. It's there when I get to hug a patient who's been to hell and back and say, *Your scan is clear.* It's there when I play my guitar and the sound is just right, and when I go home to the love of my life—who stood by me even when I was getting my ass kicked.

Like Rocky.

I was feeling a lot of that strength coming into 2020. It was a big birthday year. I was at the top of my professional game. I was healthy and knew enough to be grateful for it. I was blessed with lessons learned from parents and teachers, doctors and nurses, patients and families.

It was a moment of strength, and I was ready to get in the ring.

But it was also the beginning of a world pandemic that came along and unmoored the routines and protocols cancer teams live by. In oncology we inevitably and routinely have to make decisions in which the best we can do is choose the least bad thing. COVID-19 brought this to new and sometimes unthinkable levels for doctors and patients and everyone else involved in the medical world. Physicians asked, *Do I bring an immunocompromised patient in for blood work and risk her exposure? Do we delay a chemo session because the patient is afraid?* Caregivers asked, *Do I take my loved one who's dehydrated from chemo to the emergency room? If I do, will he then be not just sick but also alone?* People with family or personal histories of disease asked, *Should I postpone my annual screening for 6 months? For a year?*

Everyone I know who works in medicine has been impacted in some lasting way by these changes. We're all learning, even those among us who thought we had this oncology thing figured out. We will get stronger and smarter, but we will never be the same.

Again and again in this time of crisis, I've thought of two strong, smart, fierce women who continue to shape my understanding of what it means to live with purpose.

The first came into my life a few years ago with purple hair and bright eyes and the onus of living with metastatic cancer and knowing she had something to say about it that was worth sharing. The second is, as I write this page, schooling me in something I thought I already understood: courage.

Each of these women received a devastating diagnosis and transcended it. Janet did it by becoming an oracle. Alicia did it by becoming a warrior. In my life their stories lead one to the next, and in my practice I share what they've taught me day in and day out.

They are my pandemic mentors, giving me the tools I need to connect to each patient from a place of truth and love.

♡

Dr. Janet Sollod was a pediatrician, a hiker, a rock climber and snowboarder, a beautiful human being. She was also a cancer patient for nine years, metastatic for seven of them. She stopped me in my tracks at a medical conference where she gave a talk entitled "Optimistically Approaching the Abyss." She opened her talk with, "Boo! You're looking at a ghost. Statistically I should have been dead five years ago."

It was enough to seize the attention of every person in the room.

Janet was an eloquent speaker, compassionate physician, and a unique advocate in the cancer community. She would look you in the eye and tell you she'd be dying of liver failure in the near future, defying anyone to interfere with her speaking the truth. And then she would proceed to recount the things she'd been up to in her life between treatments: hiking the John Muir Trail, climbing Mount Shasta, snowboarding, dancing, and devotedly participating in a support group for young women with metastatic breast cancer—the one place where she could share her full experience and know she'd be understood.

There is power in getting patients with metastatic disease together, in facilitating a time and place where they can bring out the heavy baggage that comes with a life lived while death is standing in the corner. There are a lot of these people—in my practice alone and around the world. We are in the middle of a transformational moment in oncology when greater numbers of patients than ever are living with stage IV metastatic disease—not just for a few weeks or months, but for stretches of time that defy measurement by one- or five-year survival. I wish I could say this is a majority. It is not. Right now I have to settle for saying the numbers are growing, that there are far more of these Stage IV thrivers than can be explained simply by calling them outliers and exceptions. Much of the credit goes to new treatments that attack cancer through unique mechanisms—shrinking it, starving it, isolating it, preventing it from further growth. Some goes to improved surgical and radiologic techniques that allow us to eliminate tumors we once could not safely reach or remove.

A good oncologist spends a lot of time helping patients "surf" available treatments, riding one for as long as it is useful, then catching the next wave. With good timing and a little luck, some patients are able to push back their cancer with one treatment, then another, and another—established chemo protocols, targeted surgery and radiation, and emerging treatment clinical trials. As treatment progresses, sometimes we have to stop and do a quality-of-life check. *Will this make me feel better? Will it give me more time? Will it cause me to suffer? Can I have it near home?*

Are there good days ahead?

I meet people all the time who tell me the outer limits of the prognosis they were given by someone in the medical community have come and gone, that it's been years, even decades. Many are patients for whom the stars aligned enough to time their cancer diagnoses with game-changing treatments. Some are medically inexplicable—because every case of cancer is different, and people are more than statistics.

Right now there are over 150,000 breast cancer patients living with metastatic disease in the U.S. alone. Many of them are NED (no evidence of disease) and pursuing preventive treatments to keep cancers that we don't yet know how to eliminate at bay.

It's a position that inevitably alters your life perspective.

Janet was uniquely able to talk with other cancer patients because of the combination of her personal experience and her medical background. She was informed and in the trenches, compassionate and energetic, honest and generous with her time. On what she knew would be her last recurrence, she embraced the daunting job of talking about living while dying.

She said, "Life is terminal."

It's impossible to argue that point. At 20 and 50 and 100, we're all heading for the same end. Some of us will get there faster. Some of us will see it up ahead. Some of us will arrive suddenly.

Living with metastatic disease makes it nearly impossible to ignore the universal prognosis of death. Janet wanted the people she shared her story with to stop and think, even if just for a moment, about what we each want to do with the time we have left.

♡

What would you do? I thought I was doing it. I was doing a lot of things right. But in a cosmic response to Janet's call to live with intention, a new patient came into my life in a way that challenged and energized me. Hers was a call to action.

The call came in the form of one small, strong former Marine with vivid red hair and a tattoo of Harley Quinn on her wiry forearm. Her name is Alicia, and the sheer will she has brought to her cancer treatment has been rare and powerful and beautiful.

Alicia's disease came in a form the world heard a lot about in 2020 because of the heart-wrenching death of actor Chadwick Boseman at 43 after a private four-year battle with colon cancer. The loss of the man kids all over the world saw as a true superhero brought light to a disease my colleagues and I see all too frequently in people of all ages. Vivian was born in 1930. Alicia was born in 1986.

Colon cancer is a sneaky invader, capable of growing undetected, especially in otherwise healthy young men and women. Even when something goes wrong enough that they ask for help, cancer isn't the diagnosis most family doctors and emergency room physicians are looking for at first. There are other more likely culprits for seemingly generic digestive symptoms, even when they are severe. So even though the rate of this cancer in patients over 50 has been declining for the past two decades, it's been slowly, quietly rising in the young.

The maddening thing about these diagnoses and deaths is that they are preventable. If only we're on the lookout, we can catch it early and root it out. Screening won't prevent every case or every death, but it's a solid start, and every single person who has a family history of this cancer should have their first screening while they are 10 years younger than the date of onset for their relative.

But talking about screening wasn't going to help Alicia. By the time her cancer was discovered, it had completely obstructed her colon and metastasized to her liver. The body she had strengthened with discipline and determination was in crisis mode, and she hadn't even seen it coming.

Giving young people this kind of news is the genesis of some of the most devastating moments in oncology. Often their parents are there, and sometimes also their children. You know even as you're saying the words that you are dropping a bomb on their lives, and there is no amount of love or kindness you can serve up with it in that moment that will help.

The best you can hope for is that once the blast is over you can help the family pick up the pieces.

There are days when we deliver bad news back to back to back and wonder what the hell we were thinking choosing this profession.

I've seen so many responses, so many ways people try to process this information. I have answered ten thousand questions. But when we told Alicia she had stage IV cancer, her response wasn't to ask what would happen to her, or whether she would survive, or if she would have more surgery, or chemotherapy, or lose her hair.

She didn't want to know *if*; she wanted to know *what* and *when*.

She sat straight in her chair, giving no regard to the pain I knew she must be feeling.

"I have a son who needs me," she said. "What do I need to do next?"

I had to tell her I didn't know if there was a way to change the course of the disease—a terrible thing to say to someone who would clearly do anything to survive. With the stark truth out, however, we could talk about the chance she *did* have and what it would entail.

"I have a little sister," I told her, "and I want you to know I'm going to treat you just like I'd treat her. Everything I ask you to do will come from love."

She nodded and said, "Thank you."

"If you are up to the fight," I continued, knowing this was a foregone conclusion, "let's shrink the heck out of it with chemo and then try to cut it out of the liver. I know a great surgeon. I know he can do it if we can get it small enough. You will still—you will always—be a stage IV cancer patient, but our goal is to get you to a point where there is no evidence of your disease."

And that was it. Maybe it was her training as a Marine, or her instinct to protect her son, but with full knowledge of her statistical prognosis (which was awful), Alicia *mobilized* against her cancer. She was utterly defiant of anything the disease or the treatment could do. She kept her ramrod attitude while her Mediport was inserted, while she waited for scans, while she sat in the treatment room and let a toxic cocktail—that I thought might, possibly, maybe, push back at her cancer—drip into her veins. She showed up early for appointments. Took her meds precisely as directed, setting alarms to ensure that *every 8 hours* and *every 12 hours* were not guidelines but actual facts. She made herself stay hydrated and ate vegetables and fish because we asked her to.

She was focused and determined, but she was only human.

Halfway through, she couldn't eat. Her weight plummeted. She needed IV fluids to stave off renal failure. All the while her endgame was to get to a point where she could have major surgery—insult to injury.

Even at her weakest, Alicia carried herself with the strength of a soldier. Time and again she asked, *What do I need to do next?* and followed through.

During the final week of boot camp, U.S. Marines go through the ultimate test of their stamina and strength, their ability to function under pressure, and their commitment to their brothers and sisters in arms. It's a simulation of a battle, but the suffering is real. They call it the Crucible, and it typically starts in the middle of the night. Over the course of 54 hours, in any weather Mother Earth serves up, the recruits walk more than 40 miles of rough terrain carrying about 50 pounds of gear on their backs. They ration half a day's MREs. They sleep no more than 8 hours throughout the ordeal. When they're not hiking, they fight logistical and combat challenges that feel more real as exhaustion sets in. To get through it, they have to lean on each other, share the weight, work together.

The day of her last pre-surgery chemo treatment (and there would be more after), Alicia told me it was the hardest thing she'd ever done—and she had survived the Crucible.

Here was the real Rocky. She ran *all* the steps, did all the work, pushed herself to her limits and then pushed more. Every time I suggested something that might possibly work, she said *Let's do it now.* No matter how many times her treatment knocked her down, she got up and took another step forward. She went the distance.

♡

Alicia survived her chemo, survived her surgery. Today she is NED, one of the hundreds of thousands of metastatic patients who live both with and without their disease.

I have always brought love to my patients, but working with this quiet warrior made me reevaluate how I carry out that commitment. Every patient needs something different from their oncologist. A little more encouragement, a little more patience, a little more evidence, a little more medicine, a little more time. These days I'm doing more than just reading the room. I'm asking, *What do I need to do next?* Whatever it is, we'll figure it out. We'll take it step after step after step.

CHAPTER 20

KEEP ME IN YOUR HEART

Everyone has a role to play in the healing experience.
Each interconnects with the next.
Success happens in health care when everyone feels better.
Patient first.
Then the ripples expand
Until we are all healing together.

— *DAILY DOSE*, OCTOBER 17, 2019

In February of 2020, Anna and Oscar sat side by side in my office. They were in their 40s, with two school-age children. In an affront to all logic and decency, they were both in treatment for serious cancers. Anna was my patient, and Oscar had his own oncologist across town. Despite his ongoing treatment, Oscar showed up at Anna's every appointment. He didn't say much, but he kept constant, gentle physical contact with her—holding her hand, touching her thigh, reaching around to encircle her shoulders with his burly, tattooed arm. Their connection and mutual support was obvious and palpable.

Anna had been my patient for eight long months, during which she'd undergone surgery, chemotherapy, and radiation to eradicate her breast cancer. That day we gathered to talk about what would come next.

"You're cancer free," I told her—the best words I get to say as an oncologist. "It gets a little easier from here, but I want you to be patient with yourself, because it takes time to heal."

"How long until I feel back to normal?" she asked.

"Give yourself a few months. Be kind to your body—and forgiving if you still have some 'chemo-brain' days. You'll find your new normal soon."

As they left the exam room, Anna hugged me. I extended my hand to Oscar, wishing him well in his own treatment, and this too became a hug. I couldn't have known that thanks to COVID-19, this simple, affirming means of connection would soon come to an abrupt end, that I'd be saying things like *Haven't you heard? Sanitizing is the new hug!*

In September of 2020, Anna came back for a follow-up appointment alone. I was seeing most of my patients without their partners, children, and parents during that time in deference to the dangers of the pandemic. She was quiet, but all of us were a little quieter then—probably because we shared a hard-learned understanding of just how tenuous good health is. In one way or another, everyone in an oncology office has been eye to eye with medical fragility.

Anna wanted to know if she could go back to work. She's a nurse. Her old job needed her (was in fact desperate to fill empty staff positions) and her kids needed her income. We talked about the logistics of protecting her health and the limits of energy she'd likely run up against. She nodded and said she could start part time, that the medical center was willing to welcome her with a 20-hour schedule at first.

I was worried about her, but also happy she had both the possibility of working part time and the drive to get back to her career.

Missing the man who always sat beside her, I asked how Oscar was doing.

Anna's body remained square in her chair, but her gaze dropped to the floor and her left hand drifted to the seat he had occupied beside her.

"He's gone," she said. "Since July."

The revelation left me speechless, my heart in knots over what this gentle person had been through in the months since we were last here. While Anna had been slowly, steadily recovering her health, Oscar's disease had continued a merciless advance.

The absence of the man had seemed incidental just a moment before, but now I could almost feel his presence in the room, his stocky frame, the quiet reassurance he'd exuded.

I scooted closer to Anna and extended my hand to hers on her husband's chair.

"I am so sorry," I said, and then, to the empty seat, "I'm sorry, Oscar. We love and appreciate you. We're grateful for the strength and love you gave and continue to give Anna."

What the hell else could I say? New to her post-treatment world, minding her health, rebuilding her career, raising her children, and mourning her husband, Anna was standing at the most consequential crossroads of her life, alone.

♡

The fallout of cancer is full of devastating moments like this. That's the reason we so often talk about it in terms of battles and wars, floods and tsunamis, physical and emotional trauma. The initial barrage is shocking, full of *why me* and *how bad* and *what now* . . . Next is the siege of early treatment, when tensions are high and bodies are being opened and mended, poisoned and radiated, subjected to indignities and pain. And in between there is waiting—for scans and results, surgery, chemo, hormones, radiation, and scans and results again.

In time, whether you're cured or terminal or moving forward as a lifelong patient who will continue some form of treatment for many years to come, a new phase begins. It's not so much life *after* cancer as it is life with the reality of it, whether it's in your past, future, or foreseeable present. It's the phase of *then what?*

After the initial shock and awe of a war, of any catastrophic event, we don't just step into the sunshine and slough off the violence and grief. We tend to our wounds and our wounded. We comfort spouses, parents, and children. We start sifting through the rubble, figuring out what we can salvage, what we will carry with us, what we have to mourn and let go. Regardless of the outcome, we are changed.

Perhaps the best we can hope for is that over time our shared condition, well-defined as post-traumatic stress, morphs into something else: post-traumatic growth.

This is not a Pollyanna idea. It's a reality for millions of men and women who once had or still have cancer and the people who loved them through it. It's part of the skill set with which we humans come equipped—the ability to take heartache, injury, and grief and transform them into something infused with understanding, hope, and love. That talent for recalibrating during and after trauma is integral to our ability to fully heal. It's also the impetus for some of our greatest accomplishments—things like forgiveness and intimacy, art and music.

People who work in oncology know quite a bit about this process. My life and the lives of my colleagues are inextricably bound up with cancer. Our work happens in the crisis, and the team I am privileged to work with gets this and welcomes it into their lives. But it's not an easy thing to welcome. Sometimes in the middle of a hard day, we have to call a halt, step outside, sit in the fresh air, and acknowledge, once again, that what's happening inside today is not okay. Being so involved in life and death and life-and-death decisions is not a normal workday. Swallowing everything you feel in the moment so you can try to do some good comes at a cost. We have to thank each other and love each other and know our shared experience makes us a special kind of family.

And then we get back to work. We lean into the intimacy and emotion, the joy and pain, and doing so fills us up and makes us ready to do it again.

The paradoxical relationships between pain and compassion, suffering and gratitude, weakness and strength endlessly demonstrate that hardship opens us up not just to misery but also to perspective and possibility. If we allow it to, hardship can make us mindful of our "Here Comes the Sun" moments—eager enough to revel in them, generous enough to share, wise enough to know that even within the framework of illness or grief we still have reason to hope.

♡

How do you achieve growth during, or after, cancer? And when? Just like every other life experience, you take your own path and do it in your own time. There is no playbook, and there's no conformity required. After caring for thousands of patients, though, I can suggest a few guideposts to look for along the way.

Unburden yourself a little. Too often I see patients who carry their cancer experience like a secret—tucked into a pocket, weighing them down. It's a natural inclination, especially if you endured physical changes during treatment that stripped away your privacy. You don't owe anybody access to this truth, but please find ways to share the load so it doesn't get too heavy. Loneliness, anxiety, and self-consciousness can all accumulate if you don't have an emotional outlet.

Choose a friend, family member, or support group and make a point to talk about what you've been through and how you're feeling.

Give your fear a minute. The whole world is already afraid of cancer, and after you've gotten up close and personal with it, there's a good chance you'll fear it more. Patients have told me about losing sleep in the days before routine follow-up appointments, and about becoming so distracted by the fear of recurrence that they can't focus on work or family. How can you get past your fears? Start by giving them a slot on the calendar. Preoccupation with trying *not* to think about something is all too often a trap that keeps you locked on it. Try taking five or ten minutes every day to process this one thing. I had a patient who called it her "Holy Crap This Could Come Back and Kill Me Coffee Break." During those minutes every day, she'd write a letter. Sometimes these letters were for friends and family, just in case she did eventually get sick again (which she still has not at this writing). Sometimes she'd write to me. Sometimes she'd write to her past or future self. The coffee break became a habit, and over time it became a productive slot in her day and an extensive journal.

Go ahead and get mad. If you've had your life derailed for six months or a year or indefinitely by cancer, you may have discovered that there are (well-meaning) people who are not helping when they show up with expectations you can't fulfill. Whether those expectations entail being relentlessly positive, pretending your illness is purely a thing of the past, wanting to talk about it when you do not, or expecting your involvement in things you aren't ready to do, they can be deeply frustrating. Other things that are not helping? Aches and pains. Scars. Testy digestive systems that aren't back to full function yet. Regrowing hair. Exhaustion. Gossip. Having seen thousands of patients go through this process, I can tell you that on the other side of allowing yourself the freedom to express how you feel about this is a sense of relief and clarity. But you won't get there until you can say, *I'm having a shitty day. I'm going to have a cry and maybe pull out the few strands of hair I have left, stomp my feet and slam some doors, and then have a big bowl of ice cream.* Or whatever your equivalent emotional purge looks like. You know what you need to do. Don't be afraid to do it.

Move closer to health. Regardless of whether you're cured or in remission or in long-term treatment, you and your body have had something like a falling out and it's time to kiss and make up. The steps to this are easy in theory and difficult in practice. Instead of trying to fine-tune all your routines at once and getting bogged down in details, try to achieve three small daily goals: Eat something nourishing. Spend time outside. Move your body. It sounds too simple, but depending on what you've been through, you may well be starting from near-zero. Be patient and persistent and you'll start feeling a little bit better every day.

Believe. In 20 years of oncology practice, I have had the privilege of witnessing countless acts of faith and grace. They have not been limited to any one belief system, nor any one way of practicing. They've had remarkably different outcomes. What they do have in common is a sincere and heartfelt belief in something bigger, more powerful, and more benevolent than any one man, woman, or child. Whatever your higher power, this is an ideal time to get in touch.

Create. Music was the tool that restored my faith in people, in medicine, and in myself. Part of the process of transforming pain into something, anything, else is processing it through whatever filters are most meaningful in your life. Mine were a guitar, a love of lyrics, and a determination to become a worthwhile physician. Yours may be writing, playing piano, singing, doing stand-up, baking, whittling, painting, or gardening. This time of reassessment and renewal is the perfect moment to explore a new creative outlet or get reacquainted with an old one.

Connect. Love is the strongest medicine. The bonds we feel with one another, with our friends, neighbors, and families, are the means by which we build each other up. This isn't just my observation; it's a well-studied phenomenon. We know that social environments influence the ways we function right down to the cellular level, impacting mood, blood flow, gut health, and immune response. Equally importantly, connection is another prism through which we can take the hardest things we have endured and find some solace. Helen Keller wrote, "All that we love deeply becomes a part of us." In the aftermath of a cancer diagnosis, treatment, or loss, this may be the comfort we need the most.

♡

I was eight years old when Warren Zevon's album *Excitable Boy* found its way from studio to radio and rattled a new part of me awake—a melodic id that wanted to pound on the piano, stomp my feet to a beat, throw my head back, and howl *AH-OOOO.*

"Werewolves of London" may have been my first real taste of rock and roll.

Twenty-four years later, with decades of piano lessons and guitar sessions behind me and a career in oncology just getting started, I turned on the TV late one night to see Zevon sitting next to David Letterman, talking about a cancer diagnosis, about running out of time, about having "perhaps miscalculated" by not seeing see a doctor for 20 years. Knowing his disease would be terminal in the near future no matter what, he'd chosen to forego chemotherapy and focus on making one last album.

Just two weeks before Zevon's 2003 death, when that album, *The Wind,* was released, I brought it home and listened to it on a loop. Tucked into its 11 tracks were contributions from some of my biggest rock-and-roll heroes—all of whom had pitched in to help ensure Zevon finished his last opus. Bruce Springsteen, Tom Petty, John Waite, Linda Ronstadt, Jackson Browne, T Bone Burnett, Don Henley, and Joe Walsh were all there. It was like the Hall of Fame team had turned out to have one last jam with their friend.

The last track was a stripped-down song, just Zevon's voice accompanied by guitar and drums. "Keep Me in Your Heart" was a poignant open love letter to anyone who'd ever loved or even been a fan of the man. In it he vowed that leaving someone doesn't mean loving them less, and asked the listener to remember him in the quiet, mundane moments of the everyday.

The song was and remains a masterpiece, one that fulfills its purpose of reminding listeners of the artist, of our own lost loved ones, and even of former versions of ourselves.

When I hear it, I envision patients who've profoundly influenced my life: Chuck, Clara, Roger, Ben, Flavie, and so many others. And I recall an old version of myself—the one who existed before figuring out how to do this work in a way that sustains me. The one who was sick and unhappy and ungrateful and neglectful of his family and his music.

Ironically, it was in writing these pages that I discovered that Warren Zevon had a closer connection to my mission than I'd ever known. In his last *Rolling Stone* interview, he spoke about the challenge of creating the final album as his body was beginning to fail. The method he found for pushing through was immersing himself in creating his life's soundtrack.

"When you get into songwriting, everything else falls away," he said. "That's the miracle."

♡

I would argue the miracle is even more than the song-writing and the song. It's the love that goes into it. Love of the melody, the moment, and the message; love for the person who will hear it on the other end and know it was meant for them; the love that person will carry and share.

When everything else falls away—whether you are in a hospital exam room or tucked in bed at home, whether you are sick or well, patient, caregiver, or medical professional—the love that remains is the miracle.

I've been blessed to see and feel that love in the room with every one of the patients in this book, and with thousands whose stories are not here. It's there when a doctor offers a complex treatment plan and says, *You can do this.* When a parent or spouse extends a protective arm and says, *I'll help.* It's there when a patient shows up week after week, month after month for treatment, and the subtext to partners and children is, *I will do even this for more time with you.* It's there when that patient emerges on the other side of surgery, radiation, or chemotherapy and says, *Let's go for a walk, or camping, or to see the Grand Canyon.*

It's also there when a caregiver who has dedicated months or even years to keeping their mother, father, husband, wife, son, or daughter in a nurturing cocoon through treatment and illness reaches a moment where the patient says *Stop,* and doing so becomes their last, most gracious gesture of solidarity and faith.

In the middle of the physical, emotional, logistical, and financial challenges of dealing with cancer—with any illness—the love in the room is what separates healing connection and cooperation from an empty pantomime of it.

I swear sometimes I see that love like color, feel it like warmth, and hear it like melody and harmony. It's Warren

Zevon singing "Keep Me in Your Heart" for Anna, or U2 playing "Beautiful Day" for Brittany, or Ol' Blue Eyes himself serenading Flavie as she dances across the room. It's the "True Colors" moment when Clara walks into my office after 10 years of remission—and I realize that against all odds, she's become a mother to a perfect, precious child. It's "The Message" and a djembe drumbeat for Hope, a guitar riff for Jason, and a romping piano rag for Vivian.

♡

The line between being blessed with each new day and never seeing another is not nearly as wide or solid as it seems when you're standing, sturdy, among the living. People slip across it all the time, too often leaving wasted days and carrying unspoken reconciliations and unexpressed affection. This is one of the truths you learn by default in oncology, where the life-and-death nature of the work demands acknowledgment of the life-and-death nature of daily existence as well.

Recognizing that profound impermanence means each morning is truly a new beginning after the little death of night. That new chance to live is a privilege, one we're only afforded for a finite increment of time. In recognizing it we can reframe our experience in terms of love over fear and growth over failure. It's an easy exercise on a day with sunshine and blue skies, when you're healthy and happy and everyone you love is thriving. But how often is that? For many of us—certainly for me—it's never. Someone I love is always suffering, a circumstance driven home by oncology but not necessarily unique to it.

That leaves the other days—the ones when we're coping with illness, setbacks, and uncertainty; when a friend, parent, or partner is hurting. Those are the days that truly require engaging from a place of love. It can be taking a little extra time, making closer contact, or saying something honest and kind. It can be reaching out with a joke, or a song, or a sandwich. It can be telling someone how important they are to you. It can be listening with your full attention and with empathy. It can be strapping on your guitar and cobbling together an anthem, a thing that will bond you as surely as a vow.

Each action becomes a confirmation and an affirmation, a way of saying, when it matters most, *I'm here. I love you. I keep you in my heart.*

EPILOGUE

One of the bluntest criticisms I've received since I started down the road to being the kind of oncologist who sings and dances and jokes and hugs as part of my practice of medicine is, *Why can't you just be a doctor?* It's a fair question, and I can only answer that songwriting (and all those other out-of-the-ordinary ways of connecting with patients) creates a connection that transcends the relationship that keeps doctors on one side of an invisible wall of propriety and patients on the other. Music blows that wall down. It makes me vulnerable, and it makes my patients and me co-conspirators. The ways that we conspire are many and varied—sitting knee to knee in meditation, singing "Celebration," joyriding down the highway, dancing around a hospital room, writing a song about the open road or the power of teaching—but our connections in those small, personal moments make us stronger, more effective partners as we face the phantom.

In the years since I danced with Flavie in her hospital room, I have danced with dozens of patients. I've told thousands of jokes. I have given more quick hugs while listening to lungs than I can count, and I've written over 150 songs with my patients. Some of those songs became anthems, helping patients ride out the wretchedness of chemo and shake their fists at their disease until they reached remission. Others became elegies—bittersweet testaments to those who inspired them and their beautiful, bright souls.

I believe that music, humor, and hope can transform a patient's journey through the haunted minefield of cancer, and that figuring out how to stay connected—through small gestures and big moments and the sacrifices that ensue when you open your heart to people who need you—is the best way I know to "just be a doctor." It has healed my body and saved my soul every time the practice of oncology threatened to overwhelm me. It's allowed me to continue to treat and conspire with my patients—my partners—all the while strumming my guitar and singing my song.

What you take is what you give.
It's the message of how you live . . .
A message of hope,
Never give up, nope,
On the message.

ACKNOWLEDGMENTS

Among U2's songwriting masterpieces is *One*—a track that plays out dramas of pain and suffering and nevertheless soars to the conclusion that despite our differences in this world we *get to* carry each other. The sentiment that taking care of one another is both obligation and privilege, perhaps our highest privilege, is one that's stuck with me for nearly 30 years and counting, one that helps inform the kind of man, doctor, son, husband, and father I am and want to be. I'm grateful for the opportunity to say thank you in these pages to some of the people who have been most instrumental in carrying me—through my education, into my career, in my friendships and my family, and across the vast chasm that separates the idea of a book from its existence.

First and from the bottom of my heart, I thank my patients. You honor me with your trust. You make me laugh and cry, embrace each fight, dare to hope, and love without reservation. Being a partner and advocate in your care is the most important job I will ever get to do. Most especially I thank the patients in these pages, named and unnamed, who so generously agreed to talk about their experiences and share their stories.

To my entire work family at cCARE—I'm lucky to have the partnership we share and honored to be part of a team so full of heart, energy, and wisdom. I'm thankful every day for this practice that honors our highest shared vision of care. Respect and gratitude to Laurie Frakes, Alberto Bessudo, Edward McClay, Joel Lamon, Pushpendu Banerjee, James Sinclair, Michael Kosmo, Edna Flores, Richard Just, Marti

Willey, Jennifer Coyle, Wairimu Mwaura, and Claire Moga. I am especially grateful to José Basoria, Angelica Torres, Nancy Alanis, Jenna Hugo, and Alicia Shell, my elite-force-level care team. Thank you for giving 100 percent every day in support of our patients.

I am grateful to all the mentors who took time to teach, guide, encourage, and push me to become capable and competent in my field, especially the faculty and attending physicians at the Philadelphia College of Osteopathic Medicine and Georgetown's Lombardi hematology and oncology fellowship program. In particular, I'll always be grateful to PCOM's Mindy George-Weinstein, Bruce Kornberg, Joseph Kenney, John Simelaro, Richard Pascucci, Arthur Olshan, David Henry, Pat Lannutti, Michael Venditto, Daniel Parenti, and "Uncle" Manny Fliegelman, a true compassion warrior. Thank you also to Paul Bannen, Ruby Deveras, Claudine Isaacs, Matthew Ellis, Marc Lippman, Said Baidas, Kevin Cullen, John Marshall, Naiyer Rizvi, Jimmy Hwang, Harvey Luksenburg, Craig Kessler, Aziza Shad, Kevin Knopf, Bruce Cheson, and Nancy Morgan.

I believe everyone can be a teacher on your journey, and without certain friends who encouraged me I'd have nothing but an ever-blowing storm of ideas. Thank you to the people who helped me find my way: Kevin Kroiz, Josh Apter, Scott Piro, Todd Zeldin, Marc Schwalb, Brian Berkowitz, Jon Brodsky, Andrew Lu, Andrew Cooper, Amy Schrader, Tammy Astorino, Mimi Leitner, Ellen Harner, Lyssa Goodman, Rob Rubenstein, David Rubenstein, Jennifer Liebman, Adam Berenson, Fred and Nicole Rabner, Greg and Holly Weinstein, Gregg and Rachel Diller, Adam and Kara Cherry, Warren and Jen Wisnoff, Jeffrey Melrose, Michael Reitz, Jarad Fingerman, David Helfand, David Kuo, David Addley, Jeffrey Chester, Eric and Michelle Teichberg, Seona and Michael Lisse, Andrea King, Jill Mendlen, Barbara

Teszler, Dan Golden, Scott Simon, Chris Paben, Anatoly Bulkin, Kenneth Trestman, Victor Kovner, Nadav Wilf, and Peter Hoppenfeld. And thank you to the friends who have shown me through their actions and those of the communities they lead that combining honest and positive intention with creativity and innovation can spark brilliant, far-reaching impacts: Abel James, Shawn Stevenson, Kellyann Petrucci, Gautam Gulati, Jack Kreindler, Light Watkins, Ben Gleib, Kien Vuu, Kyle Garrett, Natalie Jill and Brooks Hollan, Tom O'Bryan, Alex Jadad, Pedram Shojai, Partha Nandi, Benjamin Hardy, Ran Anbar, Julia Grace Vishnepolsky, Liana Werner-Gray, Kris Carr, Mark Hyman, Daniel Amen, and Izabella Wentz. I'm especially grateful to Michael Fishman at Consumer Health Summit for inviting me into a room full of amazing medical minds and inspiring me to transform my journey into a message; to Daniel Kraft and Exponential Medicine for helping me express my voice; and to JJ Virgin and Mindshare for elevating the concept of collaboration to an art form.

To Rudy Tanzi, rock star, scientist, and my brother in music and medical innovation, thank you for the constant inspiration and for so generously agreeing to be a part of my publishing process.

I had no idea before embarking on this journey just how many skilled, dedicated professionals it takes to bring a book to life. I'm deeply grateful to Steve Troha and Jamie Chambliss at Folio Literary Management for believing in this book and ensuring it found its perfect home; to Reid Tracy and Patty Gift for graciously inviting me to join the Hay House family; to executive editor Anne Barthel for generously and patiently nurturing this project every step of the way; to the entire Hay House team, including Marlene Robinson, Tricia Breidenthal, Nick Welch, Yvette Granados, Howie Severson, Perry Crowe, Lisa Bernier, Arya-Mehr

Oveissi, Rachel Shields Ebersole, and Lindsay McGinty, for their professionalism and support. Sincerest thanks to Jana Murphy, my invaluable writing partner. Your research, interviews, editing, and reminders to stay true to my voice and message kept me on track from start to finish. Love you like a sister, my friend.

Thank you to Ruthie Rosenfeld for being a beacon of unconditional love and Jackie Savard for reading these chapters in progress and providing valuable and affirming feedback. Your generosity with your time, energy, and honest impressions while you were in the midst of your own cancer treatment were a blessing on these pages and a benediction for their message.

This book would be an empty shell without the inspiration of the musicians, artists, comedians, speakers, and writers who gave me the will and courage to try to create something lasting. I owe a debt of gratitude to Wayne Dyer, Peter Himmelman, Janet Sollod, Caitlin Flanagan, Craig Shoemaker, Kira Soltanovich, Barry Katz, Nick Nanton, Louis Armstrong, Paul McCartney with and without the Beatles, Nirvana, Michael Jackson, Frank Sinatra, Lenny Kravitz, Andrea Bocelli, U2, Cyndi Lauper, Bruce Springsteen, Jeff Buckley, Roger Gagos, Howlin' Wolf, Warren Zevon, and every bandmate I've ever had.

Of all my blessings, I'm most thankful for my loving, positive, supportive family. There aren't enough words to express my gratitude to my mother, Rochelle, my number one supporter, who makes me feel invincible, and my father, Barry, who taught me that art and science aren't mutually exclusive and that doctor/patient relationships start with trust. Everything I've ever become or done is because of the two of you. Thank you also to my stepfather, Marty, my stepmother, Julie, and my mothers- and fathers-in-law, Alan, Nancy, Kenny, and Patricia. I'm grateful for the love from

Uncles Barry, Teddy, Ronny, Jimmy, and Marty; Aunts Sandy, Joyce, and Ina; cousins Suzanne, Scott, Jill, Ben, Samantha, Thea, Todd, and Bethany; and dear family friends Lynne Solomon, Bobbi and Ken Martini, Bev and Dan Joie, Joan Chintz and Bob Heck, Jerry and Joyce Skobinsky, Denny and Linda Tessler, Sue and Gary Katz, and Sammy Schwartz. No one could ask for a stronger support network than I have found with all of you.

Thank you to my sister Beth and brother-in-law Casey, for always laughing at my silly bits, and my sister-in-law Brittany and brother-in-law Patrick, for showing me miracles happen right at home. Thank you also to my brother-in-law Brian, for your kindness, and to the late Scott Shapiro, for the enduring legacy of love your family continues to share.

At the end of each day, I get to go home to the people who make me happiest in the world—my children, Kaiya, Tori, and Brandon, and my wife, Julie. Thank you to my precious children for every minute we spend together and for the amazing people you are becoming. Thank you, Julie, my Diamond Jewel, for everything you are and everything you do, for bringing joy and love and understanding and *be here now* to my life. I'm so fortunate to be on this journey with you.

Lastly, if you're reading these pages, I thank you. It's an honor to be heard. I hope you'll join me in bringing love to friends, family, strangers, patients, and medical professionals too. Love is truly the strongest medicine, the point at which all healing begins.

ABOUT THE AUTHOR

Steven Eisenberg is a triple-board-certified physician in internal medicine, medical oncology, and hematology. He earned his undergrad degree at Penn State and a D.O. at the Philadelphia College of Osteopathic Medicine before completing a three-year medical oncology and hematology fellowship at Georgetown University's Vincent T. Lombardi Comprehensive Cancer Center. His research publications include articles on novel therapies for cancer, and his special interests are breast cancer treatment, cancer prevention, patient engagement, and new health care technologies. Dr. Eisenberg was one of the first graduates of FutureMed at NASA's Ames Research Center in Silicon Valley. Building on his expertise in health care technology, he joined the faculty of Singularity University's Exponential Medicine program and joined the ranks of the world's top medical innovators.

Dr. Eisenberg is the co-founder of cCARE, California's largest medical oncology practice. He serves as the practice's unofficial CEO (Chief Empathy Officer). He is also co-founder of Workup, Inc., a collaboration platform for health care teams.

Dr. Eisenberg was the first recipient of the Dr. Emanuel Fliegelman Humanitarian Award, for the doctor most exhibiting highly compassionate care during residency, and he has won numerous hospital awards for his uniquely empathetic bedside manner and commitment to meaningful patient engagement. His practice of writing songs with his patients earned him the nickname "the singing oncologist" and has helped him become the most-followed oncologist on Twitter and an in-demand conference speaker. His work has been featured on NBC's *TODAY* as well as in *People* magazine, *Huffington Post, US News & World Report, Reader's Digest,* and many other publications. He is the host of *The Dr. Steven Show* and podcast.

Website: drsteven.com

Hay House Titles of Related Interest

We hope you enjoyed this Hay House book. If you'd like to receive our online catalog featuring additional information on Hay House books and products, or if you'd like to find out more about the Hay Foundation, please contact:

Hay House, Inc., P.O. Box 5100, Carlsbad, CA 92018-5100
(760) 431-7695 or (800) 654-5126
(760) 431-6948 (fax) or (800) 650-5115 (fax)
www.hayhouse.com® • www.hayfoundation.org

———

Published in Australia by: Hay House Australia Pty. Ltd.,
18/36 Ralph St., Alexandria NSW 2015
Phone: 612-9669-4299 • *Fax:* 612-9669-4144
www.hayhouse.com.au

Published in the United Kingdom by: Hay House UK, Ltd.,
The Sixth Floor, Watson House, 54 Baker Street, London W1U 7BU
Phone: +44 (0)20 3927 7290 • *Fax:* +44 (0)20 3927 7291
www.hayhouse.co.uk

Published in India by: Hay House Publishers India,
Muskaan Complex, Plot No. 3, B-2, Vasant Kunj, New Delhi 110 070
Phone: 91-11-4176-1620 • *Fax:* 91-11-4176-1630
www.hayhouse.co.in

———

Access New Knowledge.
Anytime. Anywhere.

Learn and evolve at your own pace
with the world's leading experts.

www.hayhouseU.com

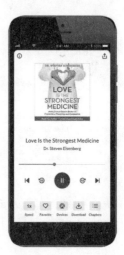